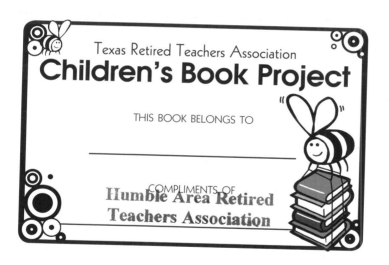

Texas Retired Teachers Association
Children's Book Project

THIS BOOK BELONGS TO

_____

COMPLIMENTS OF
Humble Area Retired Teachers Association

ASPERGER'S
ON THE
INSIDE

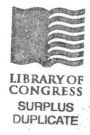

MICHELLE VINES

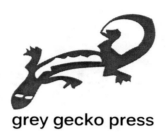

grey gecko press

Text © 2016 by Michelle Vines
Illustrations & Design © 2016 by Grey Gecko Press

Published by Grey Gecko Press, Katy, Texas.

www.greygeckopress.com

Printed in the United States of America

Library of Congress Cataloging-in-Publication Data
Vines, Michelle
Asperger's on the inside / Michelle Vines
Library of Congress Control Number: 2016935468
ISBN 978-1-9388219-5-0
First Edition

This book is dedicated to my two sons, Isaac and Trent, because as a mother, I can't help but want to dedicate everything to them.

They are my precious children and the center of my world!

ACKNOWLEDGMENTS

Eugh. This passage was hard to write, so I apologize if I haven't done it well!

For starters, I will say a big thank you to my editing and publishing team, Hilary, Josh, Jason—you did an amazing job, and the book has improved a lot thanks to your feedback! Thank you to all the beta readers who took the time to read and give me constructive comments on the book—Narissa, Kristy, Jennifer, Marie, and Jamie—and an extra thanks to Daniel, who continued to work with me after the review and has even offered to translate the book into Portuguese! Also, thanks to Alex for reviewing the advance reader copy of the book and finding all those hidden typos. You truly are a grammar nut!

Another thank you to David N. for inspiring me to want to write the book in the first place, and all the people who have encouraged me along the way. Thank you to Josh of J. P. Mitchell Photography for the fantastic photographs that were used for the author photo and to create the cover, and to the cover designer, Paulo of Maple Estudio. I should throw in a thank you to Mats Gfx for all the work he put into an alternative cover design, which, unfortunately, I did not use in the end. And finally, a big thank you to my ex-husband—"Robert" in this book—who was very proactive about encouraging me to write and who afforded me a lot of free time to work on the book.

You know I'm an Aspie and feel awkward writing the happy, fluffy prose, so please go ahead and just imagine all the additional things I should have written here!

Michelle

CONTENTS

Introduction

So, before we get going on this book, there are a few little things that I think would be helpful for me to explain first (with thanks to my editor and publisher for pointing out what a reader might be missing, or basically telling me what else I had to include!).

For starters, this is a personal story—a memoir—not a textbook about Asperger's Syndrome. So please don't accidentally buy it looking for formal information! I know for some people, having the word "Asperger's" in the title did create the impression that it may be an information resource, but it's far from that. It is a story about me—a true story, as the people in marketing like to write, but coming from a very Aspie perspective.

You'll also find as you read this book that it's very personal, with a lot of talk about feelings and relationships, particularly my relationships with other women. So if you have a fondness for reflection, psychology, and a little behind-the-scenes gossip, I think you'll really enjoy how private and juicy the book gets! But I know not everyone is into that sort of thing, so if you aren't, sorry—this book will probably have you drowning in boredom! It's a bit of a girly book, as they say. And if you hate that sort of stuff but have already bought it . . . Um . . . Um . . . Oh, look how nice the weather is today . . .

Now to quickly divert the topic to something else!

I know that I do tend to use the word "Aspie" a lot when I write. Aspie, Asperger's, Asperger's Syndrome, Autism, and Aspie again. And I guess you may find it surprising that I don't spend much time explaining these terms or attempting to pass on generic Asperger's information in the book. In fact, I make you wait all the way until Chapter Thirty-Five to even give *my* description of what Asperger's actually is, which I know—*groan, grumble, complain*—is a long time to wait!

But please bear with me in doing this, as it wasn't just a complete failure to think it through! I had my reasons. You see, for most of my life, I didn't know Asperger's even existed. I grew up with the premise that I was perfectly normal, with a just few quirks and differences to my personality. Okay, perhaps quite a few then, but they were nothing outrageous! So I always assumed that it was personality-based and I was simply unique. No one ever told me that I had a syndrome!

So when I first thought about sitting down and writing out a list of typical Aspie behaviors, I recoiled at the idea of presenting myself that way, because I really didn't want to be branded as simply someone with a "syndrome." I wanted a chance to first come across as me. No lists of signs and symptoms, no typical Aspie behaviors charts, just me.

And so, that's the journey I want you to take with me when reading my story. I want you to see that I'm a real human with real feelings and not someone you would dismiss as lacking in real emotion or ability. And in many ways, I hope I'm still relatable as somebody you could understand and even share some experiences and feelings with, which is why I made a decision early on to let that information just trickle out in bits and pieces as you read through each chapter, in a manner more true to how I came to learn about myself.

Now to please all those who want everything to be strictly accurate. Yes, from 2013, Asperger's stopped being classified as a syndrome of its own and is now classified as part of the Autism spectrum. So technically, using the term is now incorrect. But you know—details, details! I still like to use the terms Aspie and Asperger's anyway, because they're the terms I most relate to.

Anyway, moving on . . . Another thing you will probably notice about the book—if you haven't already—is that my style can be rather quirky and unconventional at times. In Chapter One, I wander into a weird discussion about why I laid the book out in question-and-answer format. And as the book progresses, I do address the reader—you!—constantly, which I hear is a literary crime known as breaking the fourth wall. Yes, I admit it: I am a serial fourth wall breaker. But I usually do it for one purpose or another, even if that purpose is often to just insert some (really bad) humor!

You may also notice that the book takes place over about a year, in which time my attitudes and perceptions change quite a bit. So please understand that at the start of the book, all the uncertainty and insecurity I convey is just reflective of the stage I was at, and my outlook does mature and become more positive over time. And as I learn and grow, I give you a lot of insight into my thoughts and feelings, so hopefully, you get a real peek into what was going on in my head as I slowly came to understand and accept my diagnosis.

Oh, and one more thing before I forget. My editor, Hilary, suggested I should warn you about my tendency to use Australian-isms. I was born in Australia and moved to the USA at age thirty. In fact, at least half my story is set in Australia, so please forgive me if I still tend to use the odd bit of good ol' Aussie slang.

My editor said that in some parts, the slang made her laugh. For example, in America, apparently, people don't talk about putting babies in capsules.[1] Really? I don't see why not. But for the sake of me not getting hauled off by Child Protective Services, we've provided translations wherever I'm told it's necessary . . . like that one that just popped up then. Great!

So please read on, and I hope you really enjoy my story.

It's so cool that you're reading my book!

Michelle

---

[1] A capsule = A detachable infant car seat

Some names have been changed to protect the privacy of certain individuals and institutions.

LETTER TO A FELLOW ASPIE

11/26/2011

I liked the phrase "meaningful meanderings" that you wrote in the previous email. It sounded a bit like poetry. The email got my mind wandering about the point of life, wealth, and living here in Texas. It's so funny that I now have this "American dream" with the house and the kids and enough money to be happy—as taboo as that is to mention. It's the sort of dream that many people work for and think is the ultimate goal. But to me, money has never been about spending. I've always seen it instead as my get-out-of-jail-free plan to not have to work again, as strange as that may sound.

In theory, if you save enough money in the bank, you could live off the interest, and that is my idea of how I could reach freedom. A life in which I could never again be forced to do something that made me feel so bad. A freedom to always be at least "okay." In the meanwhile, I'm just sort of "meandering" life because I can't find a place (a niche) that works for me.

I had so much potential once. I had scholarships through high school. At university, I won a prestigious summer scholarship at the University of Queensland and graduated from the University of Melbourne in the top 3 or 4 percent of chemical engineering students. I have bachelor's degrees in science and in engineering. I worked so hard to reach my goals and achieved outstanding results. I was driven. The world was my oyster, and I really felt like I was heading somewhere back then . . .

But that was then. I'm not exactly sure why I went nowhere.

Sometimes I think that something really special is there in me, still. I daydream about all the things I could be. But somehow, I've lost it. And I honestly don't know if I will ever find it again. Work hit, and it didn't work for me in a way that I can't even explain. All I know is I can't ever do that again. I don't ever want to feel that way again. I don't think I could keep going if I did. So that circles back to the idea of living off money.

I'm waffling here, but I think you are so much like me that you will understand my meaning. You seem to have found a little niche and a way to wander through life that has meaningful things in it for you. I'd like to find that too. Something that makes me want to wake up each day and get going.

I mean, looking after my kids is important, and I would never stop doing that, because they need me to. I think I am a great parent for them. So I'm not complaining or saying my lot in life isn't important. I was just thinking going down the track how nice it would be to find some of these little things that are meaningful to me, for ME. Not for someone else's sake or to impress or appear to be doing the right thing. Until then, I'm just wandering and sometimes looking for little things that make me feel alive.

But it's been good. Somehow, talking to you has momentarily snapped me out of thinking about the little things and viewing the big picture as it sits now. Sorry about the long train of thought. For some reason, I feel I can talk openly with you. I don't really write stuff like that to people usually.

Michelle

CHAPTER ONE

LOOK AT ME, TRYING TO WRITE!

This morning, I'm excited! I just had a breakthrough and figured out why my previous attempts at writing down my story hadn't worked! You know, those grand "lightbulb-on" moments when suddenly, everything makes sense. The "I can see clearly now!" "My perspective has completely changed!" adrenaline-running-high moments. Okay, well, maybe I'm exaggerating and it was really just a small breakthrough, but it feels pretty exciting to me. My sudden realization was . . . my writing was no good because at the time, I was angry!

I'd wanted to write a book and explain to all the people who had ever mistreated me why they were wrong and why they'd misunderstood me. I wanted to emphasize how we need stop judging each other and focus on celebrating each other's talents and uniqueness instead, eccentricities included. Every person has something special to bring to the table. Empower people and encourage them to focus on their strengths, and imagine what we could do . . .

But in my hurry to get to the parts I was upset about, my story didn't flow and make sense. It was missing too many of the positive and beautiful things that also make up me, as if trying to construct a building without first laying the foundations. I have so many better things to say—insights about the world—than just what I'm feeling frustrated about at the time. I needed to stop rushing to get to my point.

I know that for me, even when I'm at my most calm and thoughtful, getting words out has never been easy. I am in no way a writer (I say as I sit here writing a book!).

Rather, my mind is a tangle of concepts so interlinked that I never know where to start or how to get one idea out without detouring off onto explanations of twenty other related topics. I think in pictures. Wonderful pictures. Not these *words* that most people seem to love so much. So this attempt at writing, for me, is really rather a form of insanity.

But fortunately, I do know that communicating becomes a lot easier for me when I'm asked specific questions. That way, I can get on to boring people with the details straight away—the Aspie way—instead of having to wander through small talk first! So I was thinking maybe I could do something unconventional here and write this book as a random collection of questions and topics instead. It's not the way books are usually laid out, but hey, the book is about me. It might even be more fitting if it does turn out to be a little "outside of the box," not unlike myself.

Anyway, getting back to my moment of excitement, the point I was making was that maybe if I stop trying to say everything at once and instead just write a bit about a specific topic each time, I can let these thoughts of mine slowly unravel on the page slowly, calmly, and in any random order as they will. And maybe then I can get this great picture in my head to slowly paint itself into writing. *Slowly* is the key.

So that's it. I'm going to try again, this time with a lot more direction and clarity.

Wish me luck, and fingers crossed that I won't get so stuck this time around. It's time to let the questioning begin!

CHAPTER TWO

REFLECTING ON MY CHILDHOOD

So my first question is:

Q: Tell us about your childhood. What was it like for you growing up?

Ah, the innocence of childhood. Well, when I dive into my childhood memories, the first comment I have to make is how little I remember in the way of people or major events in my life. Strangely, my memories are more a series of fuzzy visuals I recall seeing through that rose-colored childhood lens of fascination and wonder. It's mostly images of things. I see myself sitting in the grass or by the potted plants in the garden, working hard on my latest form of play with my head down and my long, golden hair around me. I guess I thought often about my hair. It made me feel like a princess. I see myself spinning in circles and feeling the wind in my hands.

My mum² tells me that as a child, I was contented to play on my own. I would let others join me at times, but only as long as they were willing to play my games my way. And if they weren't, I was perfectly happy to walk off. From my point of view, what I was doing in my game was all that was important, and anything else that came up just wasn't as relevant.

---

² Mum = Mom

It's interesting, as an adult, thinking back to realize that at this time, my Aspie traits were probably more distinct than they've ever subsequently been, and yet it was the time that I was the least aware of them.

My mum tells me that when I was a child, she thought other children were mean to me, and as a parent, it was hard for her to watch. I don't actually recall noticing this as much as she did, so I can't say for sure what she meant by it, but I presume it was probably about other kids excluding me or rejecting my attempts to walk up and join them. There was possibly even some name calling. I do remember being called "stare bear" a few times in primary school.[3]

I found it interesting to hear that Mum had been so attuned to it. As a parent, it seems she understood my behavior well enough to interpret it as others misunderstanding and mistreating me, whereas a stranger may have seen it the other way around, as me behaving in ways that were inconsiderate of others and alienating my "friends" (or random playmates at the time).

However, I was never trying to upset anybody. I was just activity focused. I took a lot of pride in my work and its perfection. The point of the game is X, and what's the point having other people join if they're not going to do it properly? Unfortunately, the fact that others didn't appreciate being told when they were wrong or being dismissed didn't occur to me at the time!

Sometimes, on days when I was acting particularly unusual in my mannerisms or blunt toward others, my mother would intervene in my behavior. She corrected me and encouraged me to act "right" in little ways, telling me my hands looked wrong when I crossed them in front of my body or poking me gently in the back to correct my posture. She also fussed a lot about tasks and told my brother and me when we were getting little details wrong. She didn't mean any harm by it, of course, but she was a natural perfectionist herself and overly focused on things being done her way.

Unfortunately, the criticisms made me a little uncertain about myself, and perhaps I didn't grow up with the best self-esteem—when it turned out a superior self-esteem was really what I was going to need to cope with life as an Aspie in a teenage world. However, at least while I was young and still oblivious to everybody else, I fared okay.

I had a single friend through most of primary school and then two girls who were (one at a time) my best friends in high school, and I was content with that. I liked to spend my entire time one-on-one with whomever my best friend was at the moment, playing games or, as I got older, just talking about what was on my mind. Other than that particular person—my person—I had no interest in what the rest of the world

---

[3] Schooling is organized differently in Australia. Primary school is Prep (US Kindergarten) to Grade Six. Secondary school is Year Seven to Year Twelve.

thought of me socially. In fact, I didn't tune in to the other people in the world at all. They were just background.

I was fortunate to be able to complete my schooling in Melbourne, Australia in some beautiful little schools with impressive gardens and a lot of natural bush[4] area in which I could roam. I think I spent a lot of time just sitting in private areas of the grounds, looking at whatever live things I could find buried in the grass.

I remember many years later, one of my two high school friends, Emma, telling me how my Grade Six teacher used to make fun of me over my love of the natural world. I was fascinated with plants and leaves, bugs and insects, flowing water, animals, new growth, and pretty much all things green. Emma said that the teacher had subtly made mocking comments in front of the class on several occasions. I can't remember even noticing her do this.

On the other hand, I can't complain, as it was the same teacher who gave me good grades and recommended me for a scholarship through secondary school. She said I had a creative mind and was going to write a book one day, to which I thought, "Not a chance. I hate writing." Which is rather ironic as I sit here writing this now.

As an adult trying to think back and scan through early childhood memories for interesting or "Aspie-like" incidents, I realize just how little of my interactions with those around me I even recall. It's funny how little I paid attention to the social world then, when I'm so acutely aware of it now. But I guess it simply wasn't my focus for a time.

One memory I do recall was an incident from Grade One. It must have made a strong impression on me for it to be one of the few things I do remember! My Grade One teacher, Mrs. McKenzie, had come up with a new system to motivate good behavior in the classroom. It was called "star of the week," and in week one, I was awarded the honor of being the first star.

That class, we were instructed to make our own cardboard placards displaying a photograph of ourselves that would be put up on a special board on the occasions that we were the star. I created mine with the square photo in the middle and yellow points radiating outward from the center so that it actually looked like a star. I thought it was beautiful.

At one point during the class, the teacher wandered over and stopped me to recommend some changes. My placard wasn't suitable to put up for some reason that I've now forgotten. My stubborn self, however, found the changes to my art unacceptable. In my head, I had an idea of what I wanted, and that was what I had created. It was perfect. The idea of changing it in any way was unthinkable.

---

[4] Bush = A natural or untamed Australian wildlife area. In this context, I mean an area overgrown with knee-high bracken, long grass, or dry, scratchy plants amidst taller ferns and gum trees.

After that, I can't remember exactly what I did or said, but something happened. I misbehaved? I don't know. I must have, because suddenly, I was no longer the star of the week. My placard was taken down. I was devastated. I felt like I was right and she was wrong, and I didn't understand why she wouldn't accept my explanations. And then, for no reason I understood, she was mad at me. It really hurt my feelings, and in the future, I made sure I tried harder not say things that might upset her.

Many years later, as an adult, I looked back on my school reports for that year.

The first semester report card read, among other points, "Michelle can be stubborn at times if she doesn't get her own way."

And the second, "Michelle has shown a complete turnaround in her behavior. She is always helpful and attentive."

I was learning. Even at that young age, I was beginning to understand that changing my behavior was going to be essential to becoming acceptable to those around me. From Grade One onward, my report cards began to show a consensus that I was a model student and, although quiet, a joy to have in the class. (With the exception of perhaps my sports classes, which I never did take too seriously, much to my teachers' dismay.)

Every year, a new Form[5] teacher would report how wonderful it was to see my confidence growing throughout the year and to see me finally coming out of my shell. The reports always shone with happiness and positivity. But I have to wonder, if my confidence was growing so much, why did they still find the need to mention it year after year? I'm guessing what it really may have reflected was the opposite.

The other memories that come back clearly for me are those about the games I used to play as a child and as a teen, because of course, those were of the utmost importance and consumed so much of my focus at the time. I made up a lot of my own games and play ideas using the standard toys and objects typically available to kids. Sometimes, the rules and constructions I came up with were so elaborate, they required me to write down pages of data and details just to play the game. But this was exciting for me to compile. My play was serious business, and I did it meticulously!

Going back to when I was younger, I remember playing with dolls a lot—not the usual girly variety of doll roleplaying games, but *my* games. I had my dolls sorted by age, from the youngest, most babyish one to the oldest, tallest, most mature doll. I would place them around the house in sequence and move from one to the next, playing "growing up" as if the dolls were all the same person. This "growing up" game was to become an emerging obsession.

I played "growing up" with people tokens from a puzzle board game. The board game people wore "dresses" to show which class level they were in but were allowed

---

[5] Form = grade level

individual colored "scarves" to identify each piece. It was necessary for when I needed them to do things one at a time. I had strict class schedules, and when they got old enough, they would go and have their own babies. (Because, of course, from a child's viewpoint, sixteen-plus-year-olds are mature adults, grown and ready to have babies of their own!)

I played "growing up" with "pick-a-numbers," little origami pieces that you open up in one of two ways to select a number and reveal a fortune written inside. But to me, the pick-a-numbers again were creatures, so I never wrote anything in them. I spent great amounts of time folding them in gradually increasing sizes. The smallest ones were delicate and far too small to be possible to write in. Each one had to be made perfectly or they would be thrown away and started again.

And so on with little girls on birthday cards, balloons blown to various sizes, card decks, marbles, dandelions turned upside down, or any other little thing I could possibly turn into people or creatures by some stretch of the imagination.

Sometimes, the games were about more than just growing up. They were about culture and conformity. At age five, this is what people (or my objects) did—five-year-old cards went to school for flying lessons with the tens as teachers. I would line up each card one at a time and make them go through the process. At age six, it was the next step and so on.

It even went as far as breeding. At age sixteen, the girls in my peg games would be sent off to be impregnated—you know, one at a time—to have babies the next year. It sounds kinky, I know, but for me, it was more matter-of-fact. I was fascinated by the rules of culture and people conforming strictly to whatever the expectations were at the time. A perfection of sorts. I think had I known about cults back then, I would have found that idea also fascinating.

Anyway, I think you've got the picture! All these details and more, I remember twenty-plus years later, and yet I can't remember the real people who were involved in my life at the time. Hmmm, perhaps "task focused" is an understatement!

As I grew older, into my early teens, these games changed and developed more complexity in the rules. My brother and I added stickers to adjust "the Game of Life," allowing the players to marry and have children. I got heavily engaged in drawing up tables for things like what jobs the boys would be given, the money you had spent on their education, how attractive the girls were and how well they married (yes, the game was really sexist!!), the cost of house and car renovations, etc.

I also became interested in planning at about this age. Before each semester at school, I dedicated hours to guessing at and drawing up possible timetables for the coming school year, based on likely constraints—the likely number of each subject, subjects not repeated within the same day, whether the subject required single or double blocks, etc. I colored them in with a different and consistent color for each subject year in, year out.

I took an interest in vegetable gardening, and I completed stocktakes[6] on my seeds. I reviewed the expiration dates on each packet and drew up planting schedules that would use up all the seeds in time. I took into consideration the size of the garden, the position of the sun, and required plant spacing, and drew up layouts for the veggie garden each year.

I took out my bank passbook and calculated compound interest and made projections for my savings into the future. I altered the analysis to see the effects of varying interest rates. I projected how much money I was going to earn under a range of pocket money scenarios. In fact, this hobby continued well into the future.

I had no real notion that these weren't the types of games other ten-to-thirteen-year-olds were playing. That self-awareness wasn't yet a part of my personality. But as I headed toward puberty, something happened. My peers were growing and changing and becoming highly focused on that all-important social game that underpins teenage popularity. I had no interest (yet) in fashion or networking or who was "in" with who. I didn't change, and the differences really started to show.

It was around this time that I first encountered real troubles with not fitting in and being teased by others. Why were they no longer interested in lining up toys with me? These girls didn't make sense. But that's a story for another chapter.

Throughout this book, I plan to get back to my life story every few chapters to gradually build on my experiences. But in the meanwhile, I also have many other Aspie questions and thoughts on life that I'm eager to wander through, so I've decided to do a bit of both in an alternating manner. Thus, I'm going to move back to the present for now, but do stay tuned for the next installment of "the life of Michelle" when we get up to Chapter Five and I go on to talk about my high school experiences!

---

[6] A stocktake is an Australian way of saying taking an inventory

CHAPTER THREE

THE NAME OF THE BOOK

Q: So, why did you call the book *Asperger's on the Inside*? What does it mean?

Well, it's not about being in jail! Ba-dum-tsh. There's my first lame joke for the book. Wasn't it awful?

But more seriously, I came up with the title *Asperger's on the Inside* when I was trying to think of a way to describe how it feels to be an Aspie who appears very "normal" to the outside world, despite the complexities underneath. Most people have heard of that good old Asperger's stereotype: "We Aspies say whatever comes to our minds, oblivious to whether people are interested in or offended by our comments. We talk repeatedly about a few favorite topics and don't think to question others about their lives or interests."

Heck, let's take it to the full extreme and imagine that all of us have a monotone voice, unusual hair, and terrible dress sense. You can pick us out by our awkward postures and aversion to eye contact! But, of course, what people may not realize is that we're not *all* like that. We're human beings and learning creatures, many of us exceptionally bright. We do learn to blend and fit in (to varying degrees for different individuals), and the more apt among us do so extremely well.

Having only recently discovered my own Asperger's Syndrome, I find it frustrating that it's such a difficult thing to talk to people about, because it's something I really want to discuss. I wish I could just throw casual comments about it into social conversations and have people reply, "Oh, my aunt had that," or, "My sister's nephew's cousin's brother has that. I know what that is." But whenever I drop the A-word, people do react oddly. They either know nothing about it and think I'm confessing a concerning ailment or they assume it means I'm something that I'm not. Sometimes, it can be awkward and quite the conversation stopper.

I need a way to explain to people casually, "Yes, I have Asperger's Syndrome, but no, I'm not the man from *Trainspotting*. I'm the other type of Aspie. You know, the one you've never heard of! Yes, *that* one. The one that that is nothing like the stereotype." So I suppose that's what I'm trying to achieve in writing this book—to show the world Asperger's Syndrome from another point of view the best way I know how, which is by telling my personal story.

Now, before I get lost in my own little stories, one thing I did want to note about this book (which I did mention in the introduction but I'll say again) is that I *do not* plan to define or list my Asperger's traits the way a textbook would, so if you're looking for general information or a definition of the condition, sorry, you're reading the wrong book!

As a real person and not a stereotype or a textbook example, my personality traits are so complex, even I have a hard time determining where my personality ends and my Asperger's begins. There's no such thing as the Aspie side of me and the normal side of me. There's just me! So I'm intentionally going to leave that line blurred.

But what I can do is tell it all—the positive stuff, the embarrassing stuff, and even the personal little secrets I wouldn't normally say out loud—and let you decide what to make of it. It works out better that way anyway, because you're in a better position than I am to know what's usual and what's different about my behavior. I think everything I do is normal! So you be the judge, and perhaps when you're done, you can tell me what I've written that sounds odd or funny. I would be amused to hear it!

So, I guess I should explain, then, if I'm not like the Aspie stereotype, then what sort of Aspie am I, and how does Asperger's affect me? It's a topic I always find complicated to address.

I guess, firstly, I have to confess that I have quite a *lot* of Aspie traits buried down there where people can't see—more than I sometimes even admit to myself!

I'm the sort of person who feels overwhelmed in crowds and can find dealing with other people exhausting. I'm a little stubborn—well, okay, very stubborn—and sometimes struggle to let go of really, *really* wanting to do everything my way. I also frequently get so lost in what I'm doing that I can forget to notice and thank those around me—a bad habit, I know.

But, of course, if you were to see me out and about, these aren't the things that would stand out about me, especially upon first impression. I'm also friendly and polite, and I smile a lot. I can make small talk when I need to and fit in well enough in a crowd, and I have an almost charming way of saying odd but amusing things at random times.

You see, I've been around people thirty-something odd years now, and I did eventually learn how to temper my behavior, "eventually" being the operative word there! After having enough bad social experiences growing up (the Aspie way), it was natural for me to become a little obsessed with people-watching and figuring out how others tick, which I hear is actually not uncommon in Aspie circles!

I wanted to quote a friend of mine, Bruce Horst, here, because I think he put it well:

"We who are on the spectrum are often accused of being unaware of what others are thinking or feeling, but often, this results in us figuring out the patterns to read people. Aspies often get very good at this. It's almost a super power!

"This allows us to read between the lines in certain situations, sometimes inaccurately, but most often very accurately. It's like we have x-ray vision that lets us see into the [human soul][7]."

And I love this quote, because I think describes me to a T.[8] As someone who is just fascinated by why other people interact the way they do, I can't stop analyzing and finding the patterns in people's behavior. Even lying in bed at night when I ought to be sleeping, my mind is often ridiculously active, running over the goings-on of the day.

Go to sleep, Michelle. But what was so-and-so feeling to do and say X? Why would she say that? Go to sleep, Michelle. Oh, maybe she was thinking Y. But would she have said that if that were the case? Go to sleep, Michelle. You'll regret this in the morning!

But I can't turn it off. It's like an itch I have to scratch. My obsession. And it's such a great one, because it's the thing that has allowed me to understand others and fit in as well as I do. This *is* how I function. So despite the insomnia, I love that my mind does this.

So, you might ask, if I've become good at fitting in with people nowadays, as I keep saying, then why do I even need to mention Asperger's Syndrome? Isn't it no longer a consideration?

But that is where people misunderstand. It's not as simple as that.

---

[7] Other people's emails and letters are presented unedited.

[8] To a T = exactly, right down to the little details.

Even if I could perfect all social interaction and have it down to an art, I will never think the way a neurotypical[9] person does. My brain just processes everything so differently. This can allow me to do some fantastic things. I'm certainly blessed with more than a few Aspie talents, which I will definitely talk about later. But "the gift," as one of my Aspie friends likes to refer to it, also has some downsides that others don't see, the things that are happening on the inside.

For example: Boy, can I get exhausted from all the mental effort involved in staying socially aware! Every time I talk to more than one person at a time, every time I talk to someone when there are things going on in the background, every time I deal with strangers (whom I've not yet learnt to read), it's an intellectual effort which I can only sustain for so long. Yet in a typical workplace, this is something people are expected to do all day long.

I can be overstimulated by lights, sounds, trying to process too much information at once, etc. Lots of things I encounter frustrate me. I have a need for an orderly, calm environment, and every time someone forces me to deal with things differently (their way), I have to suppress frustration. I find other people's methods of doing things haphazard and stressful. Even just having to think all the time about which words are the right ones to say so as not to offend others—it's so tiring!

There are also serious emotional consequences to having to be so in control of one's behavior. I hate that I spend so much time pretending to be something that I'm not. It really dulls my personality, and I feel boring and unremarkable whenever I get stuck in an unfamiliar group. Some days—usually after particularly tiring events—I can get frustrated about how I came across as such a nobody. I stand there. I'm awkward. I don't really talk to anyone. Sometimes, I hate that side of me and wish I could make myself go away, as impossible as that is.

I want to be someone who is lively and relatable and connect with others in a way that they'll like and remember. You know those people, with big, alive personalities. But so often, I just can't break out of my unease and think of appropriate things to say.

I remember describing to a fellow Aspie online once how I can get trapped in an awful downward spiral. I have days where I feel sad that so few people love me and accept me for who I am, yet I don't show people who I am, because I know it won't be acceptable. It's self-perpetuating.

---

[9] Neurotypical, or NT, is a term people in the Autistic community have adopted to refer to those who are not Autistic. From my point of view, of course, I don't mean it as an insult or an attempt to create any sort of "us versus them" mentality. But it is useful sometimes to have a way to denote someone who does not see things the way an ASD individual does, so may behave differently or have a harder time understanding our viewpoint.

To the few people in my life who have gotten to know me better on a one-on-one level, the "real me" does start to emerge. I'm quirky, playful, and very cheeky. I make mischievous comments and have fun with people. I see beauty in the things around me and believe in kindness and compassion toward others. My motto could be, "Seek first to understand before you judge." I won't engage in lying, manipulation, or meanness, regardless of what the people around me are doing. I refuse. Openness, honesty, and kindness is my only style.

There are so many things about me that most people don't see. I'm drawn to the natural world—the bright green of new leaves, the sound of water flowing over rocks, a beetle climbing up a tree, the bark, the patterns in its wings, the joy of taking a walk in the evening once it has started to get dark. I pick out little obscure notes in a song and immerse myself in the melody, forgetting the world around me. I'm idealistic.

I wish this side of me could shine and I could say to the world, "Look. This is who I am, and some of it is magical." But I don't know how to convey it to a neurotypical crowd. Being an Aspie is so much of who I am, but to the neurotypicals in my life, it's a secret I carry with me. I am neurotypical on the outside and Asperger's on the inside, something I still have no idea how to reveal.

Chapter Four

Delayed Emotional Responses

Now, for a much more random topic, here's a train of thought I had one day about us Aspies and our weird emotions. And just to warn you, I'll probably throw in the odd train of thought here and there in whatever strange order they pop into my head, so please accept my apologies in advance if some chapters come a little out of left field! It's how my mind rolls.

> **Q:** Why do Aspies always seem so stoic? You look so blank when I would expect you to be crying, hugging, offering comfort, anything! Do you even have feelings the way the rest of us do?

Wow. Oh dear. Yes, I know we Aspies can seem a strange bunch when it comes to responding to drama or emotional news. I've had moments where I'm sure I looked blank when I know I should have been showing deep concern in response to something or where I even wanted to laugh at first until I realized something was really *not* funny (oops). Yet all I could muster at the time was an overwhelming self-consciousness about what my face was doing!

But I can assure you that any time we do look out of place in that heated situation, we're not really as absent as we appear. We're there, and we're taking it all in. It's just that sometimes our emotions can come to us in confusing ways and can take a little time to decipher.

I know when I have an emotional moment, I often find myself in this odd state where I'm so overwhelmed by feelings that all I could tell you on the spot is whether it's negative or positive. I have no idea what this gut reaction actually is or how I should respond to it, just that *something* is overwhelming me. So I can find myself stuck like a deer in the headlights at these times, dumbfounded by the intensity of it.

Perhaps a large part of the problem is that feelings come on too strongly for me to interpret when they first hit, and I need to step back from the situation to calm down and process it clearly. To other people, I probably appear to remain a little too un-moved, but underneath, I'll be scratching my head trying to figure out where on Earth these wild, irrational feelings are coming from. For that, I need time and peace and quiet to think.

Given enough time to ponder, however, I usually do manage to make sense of what my feelings have been. I personally have funny little ways of working through my emotions to try and force some sense out of my own brain. Do I feel more when I think about the person saying *this* line or *that* line? If *this* happened as a consequence, would it upset me? Oh, is *that* what I was worried about? Is that what was really bothering me? Until sixty-three and a half hours—and no sleep—later, I'm finally ready to respond! "Intellectual processing time complete. Please check back in now."

But, of course, by that point, it's far too late. Everyone else left hours ago!

And as much as it may seem odd after all my joking around the topic, often, several hours after an event, I can find myself quite distressed and badly in need of someone to talk to. My emotions—especially sadness and depression—get extremely heavy. Not heavy the way a typical person would feel, but the particularly hard-hitting Aspie version (intensity times ten).

So it's unfortunate that people often walk away from Aspies assuming the oppo-site of us. They see us looking unresponsive at emotional times and make assumptions about us being cold or unsupportive. They assume we're poor friends or partners—un-feeling, perhaps. But that's not what's going on at all. We do have feelings—extremely intense feelings. Sometimes it just takes time.

CHAPTER FIVE

SENIOR SCHOOL—PART ONE

So, going back to my story . . .

When I left off talking about my childhood, I was discussing how bullying and the difficulties I've had with fitting in were never big issues for me until I hit my teenage years. Thinking back on my more happy childhood times, I'm actually surprised I was left alone to the degree that I was, because let's admit it: my play was quite unique, and you would think young children would be the worst at taunting and pointing out differences in others.

However, it turns out—well, at least according to my random internet browsing—that for children on the spectrum, this is actually a common pattern, and it's often during the teenage years that a person's Asperger's behaviors can become more pronounced. It's not because we actually change in any way, but—on the contrary—because our peers around us hit puberty and *they* start to change their own behaviors and modes of dealing with each other.

It's around those years that teens start to adopt more complex social interactions and choose different friends to meet different needs. Girls in particular learn to remain positive and friendly even when they're feeling negative things inside. They start caring about social status and how they appear to others. So sometimes, passive-aggressive behaviors arise in the place of direct confrontation.

Those of us with Asperger's, however—surprise, surprise—usually don't change and tend to remain childlike in our views of life and styles of friendship. Some refer to it as naïve, but I would prefer to think of it as a type of innocence. I have no interest in competing with those around me, overtly or covertly. I just want to be myself and love the things I love and be happy for those around me when I see them being themselves and having successes too. I want to cling to one person and have them as my very close, important, only friend.

Call me crazy, but I actually think this failure to mature in this way is a good trait in some regards, and I like the way I see things. But, of course, I would say that, coming from my own idealized, simple view of the world!

So, come my high school years, I think this shift of attitude around me is what I experienced. I sat there watching my friends grow and change in ways that I thought just made no sense. I continued to want just one or two very close and intimate friendships, but my closest friends stopped wanting the same and became more interested in mingling in the bigger group.

Some of them adopted different mannerisms that, to me, looked a bit false and occasionally even mean. They changed their topics of conversation to boys and fashion and small talk in general. Why they would want to change that way was perplexing to me. But they changed, so I had no choice but to accept it and follow.

But anyhow, that's enough generalizing from me. It's time to go back and start at the beginning of my story . . .

My senior school years,[10] or what I would refer to as them, started early when, in Year Six,[11] my mother decided to move me from state school to a more prestigious private girls' school to see how I fared. My brother had just won a scholarship to a private boys' school in the area, and I think she was enjoying the happy thought of us all attending nice schools—if it were financially possible, that is. But luckily, by the end of the year, I was awarded a scholarship to continue on at the school, so that's how I came about attending high school years at St Agnes's senior campus.

At St Agnes's, I met Monique and Emma, my two close high school friends whom I mentioned in the early chapter about my childhood. We spent all our free time together during our recess and lunch breaks playing elastics[12] and hopscotch and creating our own versions of games, as kids tend to do. We had fun.

---

[10] Australian senior school = Years 7 - 12

[11] Year Six = American sixth grade

[12] Elastics is a game that was popular in Australia at the time I was in late primary school. It's similar to jump rope, except instead of swinging a rope, the players hold elastic loops in place for the other player to jump over in a special sequence. If you passed, the elastic would be moved higher and you would try again until you failed.

The three of us formed a bit of a friendship triangle, so usually at any one time, one of us was more on the outside while the other two were close, which didn't bother me that much as I just went on playing with whomever was paying attention. However, I think in hindsight that it did bother the other two, who continuously sort of competed to be one of the girls on the "inside."

One day, many years later, I remember Monique expressing that she thought we (and Emma) were really only thrown together as friends because we were the oddities who didn't fit with anyone else, and I was surprised to hear that, because I'd never viewed it that way or noticed any lack of popularity at the time. But I wouldn't have, would I! I was rather oblivious to the social world at that age. They were simply the people who sought me out, and however it came about, I was perfectly happy to just play with either of my two closest people. How would I have known if they were "weird"?

When I first arrived at St Agnes's in Year Six, Emma was the person who befriended me first. We enjoyed each other's company but had a less stable on-and-off sort of friendship. From time to time, she was offended by me or my views and comments, and in turn, I was regularly impatient with little things she did that I found wrong or inconsiderate. As a teen, I didn't have much tolerance for people not behaving "the right way," which I see now really just translated to "my way," and I could be rather blunt about it. Emma was highly sensitive and conscious of the social dos and don'ts. But somehow, we held it together regardless—well, most of the time.

I remember one more serious fight occurring one afternoon when I observed Emma standing around with her blouse bunched up around the front of her tunic in a peculiar way. I told her a little too flatly that she looked pregnant. I mean, she sort of did, with the material bunching out the front. As a larger girl, Emma had always been body conscious and didn't take this remark lightly. I believe the period after that was the longest amount of time that Monique and Emma were best friends and I was the one on the outside!

Emma, unfortunately left the school at the end of Year Seven, and after that, it was just Monique and I who were left behind.

In contrast to Emma, Monique and I actually got along quite well. She remarked to me one day how she'd always admired my black-and-white way of thinking, so I guess that was the basis for her going along with whatever I wanted, making her the type of friend who was easy for someone like me to tolerate! As an adult, I've come to understand that Monique's teenage life was complicated, with her parents going through a messy divorce and her father no longer being in her life the way she wanted him to be. She was dealing with a lot of rejection. I don't recall ever realizing this as a child, unfortunately.

Monique and I spent a good deal of time wandering sections of the school that were unfrequented by other students. The school had acquired an acreage of land next door that was, at the time, unkempt bush land set aside for future development. It was out of bounds for playing, of course, not that that stopped us! We would find piles of bones belonging to kangaroos and wallabies and a variety of plants, scrub, and interesting bugs. Sometimes there were rabbits or birds or other little visitors. Mounds of dirt made up hills for us to climb up and down. As far as I know, no teacher ever noticed us going there.

Another place where we would often spend our lunchtime was the old drama room, which was always left unlocked, attached to the back of the school hall. I'm pretty sure the drama room was out of bounds also. We used to creep in when nobody was looking and, as far as I know, got away with it. Sometimes we would be lucky and find costumes or props or other interesting things left from the classes beforehand to entertain us, but we were always respectful and put things back afterward. We weren't exactly the rowdy, destructive teen type.

The drama room had a door at either side that opened up to the backstage area of the hall stage. Between us and the stage hung long, drooping, black curtains, which provided us with hours of amusement and mischief.

I remember one day, the choir was rehearsing in the school hall, standing on some pews such that the conductor's back was facing the stage. Monique and I devised an amusing idea and spent the first half of lunchtime giggling and running around the school collecting sticks, twigs, and plant parts from the garden beds. We created a little puppet head out of a rose seed and thorns and leaves, which we poked through the curtain to simulate a face looking around the stage. We may have stuck our legs through the curtains too, for all I remember. We heard laughter from the choir and ran away fast out of the back door of the drama room and were never caught.

I guess I was a bit of a serial rule breaker so long as the chosen behavior wasn't hurting anyone. I felt like if I caused no harm, then logically, I wasn't doing anything wrong.

I suppose, in hindsight, it must have seemed odd to the other girls at the school that Monique and I spent all our time sneaking off alone. For me, it was anything to get away from the noisy crowds of schoolgirls, which I found extremely irritating. I had an audience of one, which was all that I needed—someone to voice my opinions to and to keep me company.

Unfortunately, Monique had to leave the school at the end of Year Nine, as she had a bursary[13] that ran out, and the school didn't intend to renew it, whereas my scholarship remained intact. I'd always been the more studious one, and I guess I kept my

---

[13] A bursary is a special scholarship for a person who couldn't afford to attend a school otherwise

grades at the point they needed to be for my scholarship to keep getting renewed. It never felt right to me, the way she was pulled away, and her moving on was a big loss. But somehow, I managed to keep my spirits up about it all and made plans to still see Monique on the odd occasion after school and on holidays. We intended to stay in touch, at least.

As the summer holidays came to an end and the new school year approached, I started looking forward to attending class again. I did like school, after all, and just assumed I'd go about my business the way I always did and new friends would stumble into my path. This year—Year Ten—new friends were going to be on the top of my agenda.

So it wasn't until that next year, without Monique by my side, that I actually noticed for the first time that things weren't going to be as easy as I'd thought. I walked in that first morning ready to socialize with the girls in my classroom, and I made an effort to look at and talk to them properly—the girls I'd failed to notice before. I tried to tell them about my interests and get to know who they were. I walked up and stood with them to join in on conversations, and that's when I really saw it. I saw what Monique had noticed all along.

Somewhere in time, unbeknownst to me, I'd become unpopular. I'm not exactly sure how it happened. I thought I mostly got along with everybody—well, as much as I cared to acknowledge them anyway. Maybe that was the problem.

Then another small piece of the puzzle came to me early on in the year when I discovered that a few of the girls (at my girls-only school) had circulated a rumor that I was gay. I suppose it had started during all that time I spent alone with Monique. After all, in other people's eyes, what other explanation could there be for two girls sneaking off to private places? It's not something I think should have made a difference, but apparently, it did, and the gay snarks I got when going about doing seemingly normal things were surprising.

I should note, it has certainly given me an appreciation for the difficulties faced by those who really are gay and have to go through the torments of high school. Teenage girls can be so cutting in their remarks!

Anyway, whether it was this rumor or just elements of my personality that made me unfavorable I'll never know. I just know that I was lacking that one friend I needed to confide in, which has and will always be an essential thing for me to have.

As the school year moved on, I found that lunchtimes became quite difficult for me to get through. The school had three Year Ten classrooms and imposed a rule that lunch must be eaten in one of them. I naturally tried the classroom that I'd been allocated to first, but a few of the girls in that room seemed agitated by my company.

One girl liked to flick bits of food at me and made remarks that I can't now recall. I remember finding rice stuck in my hair later one day. Another girl referenced bad smells as Michelle Stutsel's B.O. (Stutsel being my maiden name), and that was the point at which I realized I needed to start wearing deodorant! Oops, I'd just thought that was normal sweater smell. But I fixed that quickly. For the most part, I tried to just sit to the side away from them and eat my lunch in peace.

I remember one particular lunchtime when a few from this group were repeatedly flicking water at me from their water bottles as I tried to eat my lunch, and they just wouldn't back off. I was getting fed up, so I went to the bathroom and filled my whole lunchbox with water and sat back down. I told them if they flicked me again, I would tip my lunchbox over them. I guess they thought I was bluffing.

One completely soaked student later, I think I had made my point, and they stopped bothering me, at least with food and water. I think if anything, they were shocked I actually followed through! But that's me. If I say I'm going to do something, I will!

When the teacher came in for class after lunch, I remember her demanding an explanation for all the water spilled on the floor. The other girls laughed and said a few times, "Michelle Stutsel wet her pants." I said nothing. It was pretty clear that I wasn't wet. Fortunately, at the mention of me being the culprit, the teacher didn't pursue the issue any further, so I got away with the "crime."

Interestingly, this wasn't the first time I got away with something that I'm certain other students wouldn't have. At the time, I didn't think a lot of it, but it occurs to me now that maybe then, even the teachers knew I was different and took pity. They just didn't tell me that.

Another similar incident happened during art class one day. A girl in my class, Nadia, was touching my leg under the table, saying, "Do you like that, Michelle?" in a provocative tone. It was all in the theme of "gay taunting," and of course I didn't like it. I told her to stop or I would throw my paint on her. She didn't, so I picked up the paint and threw it at her, much to the shock of everyone on the table.

Immediately afterward, Nadia went running to the teacher, protesting about the paint on her dress. The teacher looked maddened at first at the sight of someone with paint on their school clothes. This was a Year Ten[14] girls' class, and paint fighting was definitely not the sort of behavior you'd expect. Her anger seemed to subside, however, when Nadia pointed me out as the culprit. I never actually got asked for an explanation, and I never offered one. I suppose I didn't talk that much back then, at least not in public. In the classroom, I was quiet and seemingly shy. The class moved on.

After that incident with the water, I didn't try and eat my lunch in that classroom again. I joined a second one in the hope that the girls would be nicer, and for a short while, I thought this had turned out fine. But then I heard the rumors that, apparently, I was visiting because I was in love with Debbie, one of the girls in the room.

---

[14] Year ten = American tenth grade

Oh, for heaven's sake! Debbie was a student who talked a lot, so it was hard not to look and listen. In those days, I think I had a slight tendency to stare and hadn't fully mastered appropriate eye contact. (i.e., look for a few seconds, then look away. Look slightly to the side. Look at people's noses, cheeks, or forehead if looking at their eyes makes you uncomfortable. Look back again and repeat, etc.) So that didn't help. To me, Debbie wasn't anything particularly special, but these rumors take off fast!

Following that, I gave up and found myself a new alternative. The school had a quiet strip of dirt beside a fence, hidden at the back of the Year Ten classrooms between the tall brick building and the fence. It wasn't much for scenery, but I found it an easily accessible place to sneak out to and eat my lunch for the rest of the year.

I was breaking rules by eating outside, but I assessed my risk of getting in trouble for doing so as low, and it wasn't completely unpleasant there. I had peace and quiet and time for my own thoughts and even a little grass and the movement of bugs and small animals out and about. But I was alone. Every lunch time, for about six months, alone. I don't have to explain to you how depressing that semester was.

I think I changed my behavior a lot over that year. It was that year I suddenly started to notice and pay attention to my peers, and with no one to talk to, I had a lot of time for studying other people's interactions. I picked up on some little rules of what people do and don't do and adopted a few more "usual" behaviors. Now that I'd taken interest, I learnt quickly and became a lot more what you would call "normal" rapidly. After all, I'm a quick study.

However, it was also unfortunately the year I started to lose my own personality and self, an unfortunate consequence of being required to act in order to be acceptable. I felt sad and alone frequently and was willing to bend more than a person should have to. I had to try so hard.

As the year moved on, the good news is that I did slowly start to find girls in my classes who were more positive toward me, and I gradually made new friends. In fact, by the beginning of Year Eleven, I'd integrated into a new social group entirely. I wasn't a core member of the group, of course, but I was accepted as a "B-lister" and included in the odd events. It was a new type of social interaction for me, and some girls were actually nice.

However, even though things were looking up for me, for many reasons, I made a pretty bold decision that year, that I didn't want to continue at this school any longer. My history and expected personality there were too set in stone, and I felt like I needed a clean slate to really be free to find myself. I wanted to start afresh around people who had a positive impression of me, and more than anything, I wanted to see my old friends again. I missed them a lot.

So, toward the middle of that year, I told my mother that I wanted to change schools to the school that Monique and Emma were now attending. And fortunately, she supported my decision. It was really very good of her to help me in this way, considering it meant me dropping a scholarship at a private school to move to a far less prestigious, government-subsidized high school. I'm not sure all parents would have been so understanding. But it was definitely a positive decision for me. And that's how I came about changing schools midway through my Year Eleven Victorian Certificate of Education.

Before leaving, things became a little strange for me in my last few weeks there, as I had difficulty telling the other students about my plans to go. I've always found it hard to make big announcements, especially the ones that bring out the most emotion, as it's so awkward for me to try and work out whose reactions are sincere and whose are not. I mean, in reality, not everyone would be expected to care, but they all say they do with hugs and kisses and "lots of love" language.

I don't know how to react to it, and I'm worried that I may not feel enough at the time to make the right sorts of expressions on my face. How am I supposed to look? Am I supposed to tear up? Eugh. The situation is awkward, and I can't stand being in it.

So in the end, I didn't say much to many of my friends and just snuck away quietly. And I suspect after I did go, that one or two of my closer friends (one in particular whom I can think of) may have felt betrayed that I left without ever telling them in person. It wasn't an intentional slight or a statement about how I valued them. I just couldn't bring myself to raise the topic, especially to those whom I wanted to care. That's always the hardest part, so I'll say sorry now to any of them who ever get to reading this!

And then that was it. My time at St Agnes's was over, and I was gone, ready to begin a brand new chapter . . .

Chapter Six

Are Aspies Selfish?

Q: So, while we're talking about being inconsiderate to others, something I've noticed is that people with Asperger's have a tendency to be selfish and insensitive to their peers. Why is that?

Wow. That's a harsh question. If I wasn't writing the questions myself, I might be offended by that!

But more seriously, I bring this issue up because I've realized over the years that this is one common way that people see us Aspies. When we bring the topic back to ourselves or our interests just that bit too often or fail to respond emphatically enough to other people's issues, other people don't just see a conversation deficit. They can also interpret it as us not caring or only being concerned about ourselves. To some, this translates to us being fundamentally selfish. Or even more than that, they may even assume a hint of sociopathy. Sociopathy! I know.

However, I would like to point out to the general public that how things look on the surface is not always representative of what's going on underneath. And when it comes to Aspies, there is a huge difference between being *self-focused* and actually being *selfish*. Allow me to explain . . .

I would say that being *self-focused*, in an Aspie way, means that we are in our own little world and are sometimes so preoccupied by thoughts about ourselves or our own interests that we fail to fully notice those around us to the socially acceptable extent.

Whereas I would define being *selfish* as being fully aware of others' wants and needs, yet choosing to put yourself first anyway.

I may be self-focused—perhaps a little more often than I should be—but I am by no means selfish. In fact, I can be very compassionate and selfless, especially when it comes to the most important people in my life, such as my family and especially my children.

So why, in my life, have people assumed the worst? I guess the answer has to do with inattentiveness and the way that people interpret that. We Aspies do have a tendency to get caught up in our own thoughts. We daydream and think about the topics that interest and inspire us. We get frustrated when others interrupt our thoughts and plans. Perhaps we fail to pick up the signals from other people indicating that they might want or need something from us. Or we don't realize the contributions that others are putting in and that we are expected to also contribute in a similar way.

Everyone is planning and decorating for a big event? Since when have I ever cared about decorations? Uh-oh . . . was I supposed to? Oh, was everyone helping out with the dishes? Oops. I didn't notice. It's too late now. How awkward. What do I do?

I know that when I'm on to something exciting, I might just be too "busy"—temporarily—to register much of what else is going on around me. After all, one of the key talents that comes with Asperger's is the ability to fixate and focus on the things we love to the exclusion of all else. It's part of what makes us brilliant.

One of my Aspie friends, Rob, recently told me that after his first divorce, his wife said to him, "You are the most selfish person I've ever met." And what was his reaction? He was fascinated. More than that, he thought it was a breakthrough. He'd never had that feedback before or realized that people saw him that way. You see, that's a big problem with the neurotypical world. Many people don't ever tell you when you do something "wrong." Instead, they treat you in cool and contemptuous ways for a while. So how are we supposed to know?

Interestingly, when you put a group of Aspies together—in my experience anyway—we don't view each other as selfish at all. We communicate directly and tell each other what we want. There's no gap between how we're expected to behave and how we understand the expectations. It makes me pose the question, is the problem really caused by Aspies, or is it more an error in communication? Namely, a failure of neurotypical people to communicate to us in a manner we find satisfactory. We naturally communicate one way. Typical people communicate another. Maybe we're just hitting a brick wall at the interface.

Regardless of the cause, we're unfortunately the minority, and it's a typical world that we live in, so we're going to be communicated to in the same way as everybody else, especially if our differences are invisible to the people around us. The other people in our lives are unlikely to even realize that we're absorbing information and viewing the world in a very different way than they are. So, sadly, they may judge us as regular people just being difficult, lazy, or selfish. But I hope this passage can at least create a little understanding when it comes to that.

So, circling back to my original question of why people with Asperger's are so selfish, my simple answer is that we're not. We're just not as good at picking up on your subtle communications and knowing how to respond the way you expect us to. But please don't interpret that to be anything more than it actually is.

CHAPTER SEVEN

HYPERFOCUS

Q: Now to move into the real nitty-gritty of what being an Aspie means. Tell me about the concept of "hyperfocus" and what it actually means to you.

Ah, I love this topic. Even the word "hyperfocus" is happy music to my ears.

Being able to hyperfocus is one of the awesome traits that I think is so key to being an Aspie for the many of us who experience it. It's both a delightful, pleasing thing when we get to become fully engrossed in something of interest, and also a frustrating thing when somebody or something causes us to have to snap out of it!

In a study posted online by RDOS[15], in fact, the statement, "I frequently get so strongly absorbed in one thing that I lose sight of other things," was one of the most agreed-upon statements by people with Asperger's Syndrome, with a correlation to their Aspie test score of 0.67. (I know that doesn't sound high, but it was the second highest correlation score out of over a thousand questions, so basically, it's high.) And the question, "Do you become frustrated if an activity that is important to you gets interrupted?" also ranked very highly.

---

[15] http://www.rdos.net/eng/aspeval/relf1.htm

So yes, it is an extremely common, if not key, Aspie behavior to become hyperfocused on a topic or activity to the exclusion of all else. And do I relate to this trait, you might ask? Yes! You have no idea how much!

When I truly focus on something, I lose myself in it to the extent that the rest of the world becomes a frustration, an obstacle getting in the way of what I want—no, what I *need*—to be doing right now. The times that I get caught up like this are not that common, but when they do occur, trying to continue with normal life creates an inner turmoil of enduring, acting the part, and trying to hold out until the next free slice of time in which I can get back to what I really want to be doing. It's all I can think about. In this particular aspect, my inner Aspie is overwhelmingly strong.

I'm known for skipping meals because I'm so drawn to an activity that I just can't bring myself to stop. I work for hours and hours on end when I have a task to complete—even something as mundane as shopping for a rug—because the thought of stopping half way is, well, unthinkable. I must list every option there is and systematically work through them to eliminate the features I don't want. If my search was incomplete, it would unsettle me. Once I start, there's no stopping. Only completing the task will do.

I know that when I go shopping with others, they can find me tiresome sometimes when I'm on a mission to buy something in particular. People tell me to stop, have some tea or coffee, take a break, sit for a while. But how can I when time is ticking away? My mission is incomplete and gnawing at me. I must go on!

Sometimes, my tasks can be long-term projects, which can be a challenge when combined with the fact that I actually have a life and live in the *real* world, where there's housework and daily chores to do and time limitations.

I'm going through a period like this now in regard to my sudden inspiration to write this book, not that I'm writing constantly. I write when I have an idea and the inspiration to do so, but it can come at the most inconvenient times. As a mum, I often need to be feeding, changing, looking after, and just giving attention to my children, and I'm not free to just drop everything and start writing as the mood takes me. So I force myself to continue with normality and act the part while the thoughts well in my head. But I'm antsy and unable to sit still or concentrate on anything else properly while ideas are flowing. Until I can write them down, they engross me.

Sometimes, by the time the chance to do that arises, the thoughts are gone and the moment lost, and I mourn the loss of those perfect, amazing, breathtaking words that I imagine might have been written. (Of course, they're only perfect like that when I never get to read them back!)

I'm just learning now how to live with the concept that it's okay if a train of thought is lost. Others will come. I don't have to capture and include everything I ever think of. It's such a new idea to me and takes patience that I'm just learning to have.

By the time this book is written, I think I'll have formulated and lost sixteen times as much prose in my head. But that has to be okay. As long as I manage to capture some of the best ideas in the end. It'll be okay. I'm trying to convince myself here . . .

Something else that's holding my focus right now is my new Aspie group that I've recently started attending and how talking to other Aspies makes me feel alive. There are so many exciting concepts to explore and the feeling of not being alone and having so much to say on a topic is stirring me to want to create. In fact, it was one of my Aspie friends who motivated me to sit down and try and write this book again and triggered that buzz of excitement about it in the first place. Thank you, David N.! (He requested his surname remain anonymous.)

I've been very much enjoying corresponding with my newfound friends via Facebook and email. It's exhilarating to be able to connect with someone on that deeper, intense level and to have so much in common.

This morning, I went to the hairdresser for a cut and color and was awfully aware that I ought to be engaging in small talk, focusing on other people, and staying with reality. But the preoccupation was too strong today. In my head, I was forming the words to an email, the next thing that I wanted to say to somebody. And by the end of my cut, I'd written this chapter in my head (of course, a little differently, as that set of words was among those lost to lack of opportunity to put them on paper).

I'm sure the hairdresser assumed I was quiet or shy. That's okay. Or did they think I was vague and a bit mentally absent? Did I look glazed over? Every now and then, I would be asked a question, and I would have to snap out of it to answer. I'd have to think about what they said, concentrate on making the right facial expression and tone, and formulate an answer in words.

Inside, it agitated me. I just lost a paragraph of imaginary writing, not that I was going to get it down anyway. But it would take me away from that soaring feeling of ideas flowing. I want to immerse myself in that. I mean, all I really want to do is go hide in a corner somewhere, alone with my thoughts and without the distraction of having to be conscious of how I look to others or responsive to their approach.

This high state of mind when I just get a new idea has thrilling physiological effects. I feel like someone who has just drunk a large amount of caffeine. I'm buzzing. It lingers longer than the caffeine would. The excitement, combined with some sort of anxiety, can make me tingle. Often, when I have these ideas, I lay awake for most of the night, unable to calm my mind. Is this unhealthy? Should I be fighting it? Who am I kidding? I don't want to. I want to stay like this forever. There's no feeling better than having something exciting and inspiring to think about. I wouldn't give it up for the world.

CHAPTER EIGHT

ASPERGER'S AND RELATIONSHIPS

Q: And now for a bit of dirt on you. Tell us about your relationships. I want to hear all the details!

Oh yeah, that topic. I was rather hoping that as I wrote this book, I could somehow avoid saying too much about my relationships, as they're a rather personal topic and not things I'm completely comfortable with revealing to the world! But it seems people just want to know.

First, my imaginary question-asker brought up the topic (You traitor! Aren't you supposed to work for me?), and then a lady I had review the book also commented that it would be a serious omission to leave these details out, as it's stuff that parents of Aspies might want to know.

So I guess I will reveal a little.

Well, firstly, for me personally, I think my relationship experiences and challenges have been similar to those for any typical person. I've had boyfriends since just after high school when I turned eighteen. I married when I was twenty-five and separated in my early thirties. And, of course, I have two wonderful children as a result of that union.

I can't say my relationship skills have been perfect or even close to it. Like everyone, I've had to learn and grow from making mistakes. When I was young and in my first relationship, I thought it was fine to regularly tell my partner their mistakes and things they can do to improve. I had to learn a bit about male pride and why that has a degrading effect! In my early-to-mid-twenties, I think I used the intensity of infatuation and male attention as a pick-me-up to pull me out of depression, and I had to realize that I could never truly be well that way, putting my happiness in someone else's hands. There are moments I would take back if I could.

But I think that's all I'll say about my own personal faux pas, as we all have our flaws, and they're not the things I really want to highlight about myself and my past.

On a more positive note (or at least something my parents would have thought was positive!), I did seem to take a lot longer than most to develop romantic interests. I just didn't care to chase boys the way the others did, and while my friends were out beginning their dating adventures, I was happy to ignore it and do my own thing.

I recall one night when I was around seventeen, wandering the beach at night with two of my high school friends, when—to my horror—we were approached by two older boys, whom my friends decided to pick up and bring back to the holiday house we were staying in. I spent the rest of that night hiding in my room to avoid the awkward socializing going on out there and was relieved when I heard that the girls didn't like them anymore and had asked them to leave. Apparently, the story was they had raided the fridge and eaten bacon fat, which my friends described to me as "completely gross." Or whatever. I was just glad they were gone.

Another time, I remember being reluctantly convinced to go out to a night club with a group of guys living in a share house with me in Queensland for the summer while I was working at the university. I climbed into their car, and off we drove. It was all a little unnerving for me, and I remember thinking, "Why did I agree to do this?" When we got to the club, however, it turned out I didn't have the right student ID card to get into the campus club, as I was an employee, not a student. And even though the last two guys saw my predicament, they went in anyway, leaving me stranded.

I called a taxi to get myself home, and I'm pretty sure that was the last time I ever let a group of people drive me off anywhere! I just didn't care enough about sex and popularity to want to do these wild and crazy things.

Now, I'm sure there are a lot more personal—even juicy—stories I could tell, such as the time I went skinny dipping and got up to mischief with my boyfriend in his family pool, only to realize later that his family had come home and could see everything out the window. How embarrassing!

But for the most part, my experiences have not been all that Aspie-specific, so I promise you're not missing out on anything important here or anything that would be of relevance for Aspie parents. I was mostly pretty boring and only took interest in getting involved with long-term friends. I took a long time to return my partners' interest, and I avoided anything wild and loud. So, out of respect for the guys I've dated, that's all I wish to reveal about my romantic life. Sorry. You can call me annoying and throw tomatoes at me now if you like!

On the topic of Aspie relationships in general, however, I think I do have quite a few useful comments I could make. For starters, I will confess that—politically correct or not—I'm so glad to be a woman in this regard, because I really think we do get it easier than the men! I know, I know, there are some Aspie women out there who have a really hard time too, especially in regard to presenting themselves and getting noticed, and I don't want to minimize those struggles in any way.

But for many of us women who do figure out with time how to play the female role and present ourselves in a feminine way, the rest is honestly not so bad! Men don't hate our Aspie personalities. In fact, in my experience, many men have seemed to like my Aspie quirks and often even find me charming or my rationality refreshing and a relief from the norm. I've received compliments about how captivating my personality is. (Although, admittedly, being nice looking probably prompts some of that too!)

When I look at the Aspie guys I know, however, I can't help but notice how quickly typical women are repelled by those same traits and how much male Aspies can struggle in want of a partner. I feel sorry for the friends I have who are left with so much longing and so little interest from the women around them. I can only imagine the frustration. I'm sure I know many Aspies who could write chapters and chapters on Aspie relationship failure stories. (I can think of one friend in particular!) But I'm afraid he'll have to write his own book on that, as I have little to contribute.

On the downside to being a female Aspie, we do have some things we need to watch out for. I would say on the whole that we're more vulnerable to being preyed upon romantically, as we tend to be so oblivious when it comes to relationship politics. I remember when I first read articles online about Aspie women being at risk, and I sort of poo-pooed it, because I never thought of myself as low functioning enough to be at risk, and it's very hard to see yourself that way. However, quite recently, I had a bit of an epiphany and realized something about myself.

Despite thinking I was so competent and on top of relationship issues, I worked out that I think I have trouble distinguishing genuine affection from being told what I want to hear, and it's taken me many years to really understand what true affection feels like. I also realized—the more shocking part—that others *can* read these subtle differences that I couldn't. As an Aspie, I guess I was just missing those signals that make all the difference between love and acting. An important difference to notice! All these years, I never knew.

On a more comical note, I've also had difficulties with coming across too flirty when I'm just trying to be friends. It's such a fine line to walk that I don't seem to realize that there are moments when I accidentally cross it. What's wrong with twirling my hair anyway? It's comforting! But in all seriousness, it can lead to problems too.

Another rather recent observation I've made is that Aspie relationships seem to be extremely emotionally intense in comparison to those of our typical peers. That probably doesn't surprise you that much, but it took a while for me to see, because who knows what's "normal" when it comes to relationships? I'm not privy to what goes on behind closed doors and what others say in their most private moments, so I find it hard to observe, analyze, and learn the way I usually do when it comes to more personal interactions.

I wish I could spy on others in private—oh, I would enjoy that so much (don't tell anyone I said that!)—but I think I would be called a voyeur and slapped on the wrist. So alas, I've had to learn the slow way by winging it, and I've only more recently begun to notice the funny little intensity differences that have slipped out in little (and not-so-little!) ways.

For example, when the excitement of a new partner hits, I've noticed how many Aspies (myself included) have a tendency to obsess zealously over them and want to see or think about them constantly. It can be a bit heavy for the unsuspecting neurotypical, especially if not reciprocated!

I was in a position a while back to observe the fallout when an Aspie friend of mine, Jason, emailed far too many contact details to a girl he was only just getting to know and messaged her several times a day. It's hard to explain to him where he went wrong and why she didn't respond to it other than to say that over-intensity makes him look like a stalker. He failed to comply with little rules like "wait until you hear from her before you text again." He told her how to contact him at every part of the day and how his routine would affect what medium he would respond to and when.

Parts of it would be almost comical except for the fact that he's actually a really nice guy and these setbacks knock him hard. I wish I could somehow convey to him exactly where that line is between enthusiasm and too much. But life is so complex and individuals vary so much that all you really have to go on is interpreting the subtleties in body language and tone—exactly what an Aspie can't do.

Another example is the intense difficulties we Aspies can have with *emotional regulation*, which I've experienced firsthand. Emotional regulation is a technical term I've seen in online articles—sorry to feed you technobabble. In simple terms, it means that when we feel an extreme emotion, such as sadness, we can stay in that emotionally extreme state for a long time with little ability to make the feelings go away.

In a regular person, heavy feelings would naturally dissipate after an event, particularly if a person distracts themselves with other things, so it's a lot easier for regular people to cope with overwhelming feelings. For Aspies, our highs may be higher, and our lows can become really distressing, because they just won't let up. It takes a bit more work for us to learn to be gentle with each other, but the good news is we do learn.

For the most part, however, other than these barriers and—you know—my personally being *completely* different from everyone I know, it's all been pretty normal for me. I'm a little amused that after discussing how little I have to add on the topic, I then went and wrote ten paragraphs on it! Oops. How very Aspie of me. I've said much more than I intended to.

So, enough of that, then. Time for the next chapter!

CHAPTER NINE

SENIOR SCHOOL—PART TWO

Okay, heading back to the story of my high school years.

After having walked away from St. Agnes's once and for all, I began anticipating and preparing for my new life at my up-and-coming co-ed senior school, Beaconhills College. I got to work (or play, for me) daydreaming and making up fantasies about how I was going to thrive and be popular in this new arena. Little scenarios played out in my head of people coming up and taking interest in talking to me, boys paying me attention, etc. In my head, I was queen of my new world.

I also grew excited at the idea of being able to see my friends Monique and Emma once again. It felt like it had been too long since I'd had any close-knit, intimate play-mates, and I was so relieved that I was about have that back. Life was going to be fun again! This time, I had learnt to value others so much more than I ever had in the past. Old, solid friends are like gold, and I wanted to embrace that.

So on my first day of school, I walked up into the office area side-by-side with my mum. She dropped me off and said goodbye, and I remember it taking a while to be seen. But after a nervous wait in some chairs outside an office, I was finally welcomed by one of the teachers, who walked me around and introduced me to others whom we ran into. I can't remember now which teacher it was or even picture her face, but I do remember that it felt unusually laid back, and I wondered, wasn't it a problem that I wasn't in class yet?

The whole culture of the school was different from what I was used to, and it surprised me in various ways. It was a government-subsidized co-ed school and didn't have all the bells and whistles that St Agnes's had had, nor did it have nearly as many rules. We were allowed to wear sweaters without our blazers—oh the liberty!—and school pins on our clothes, a look that was definitely considered too messy to be seen outside of grounds when representing St Agnes's. I no longer had to listen to excerpts from *The Diary of Anne Frank* every morning from assembly or donation speeches.

The principal back at St Agnes's had been prone to whimsy, and we often thought it tiresome. I recall how one morning, she'd given a speech in which she tried to inspire us to donate by describing two dollars as "just something you kick under the bed" and how much I had resisted that idea, thinking, "Hell no it isn't! I guard my two-dollar coins like precious gold!" It made me more determined than ever that there was no way I was giving up any of my money for the school! At that age, I couldn't possibly imagine what the school could want *my* money for.

Now, as I settled in at my new school, I could see the difference that school fees can make. There was no nice school hall with comfortable chairs for me anymore! Instead, I found myself sitting on the ground in a great grey cement square every morning before class and reciting the Lord's Prayer to start off the day. The assemblies were long and boring, and I realized that suddenly, Anne Frank didn't seem so bad! I mostly stared at the ground for that part.

I also noticed the absence of the assembly choir and daily singing and, surprisingly, found myself nostalgic about it. Though I'd been too shy to join a choir or commit to anything while I was there, the singing at St. Agnes's had had a place in my heart that I only really noticed once it was gone. It goes to show how easy it is to take the most beautiful things in your life for granted.

The addition of boys to the school was also new to me and a bit of a shock to my system. I wasn't familiar with the sexual element of having *males* around, and at first, I would blush when addressed, wondering what they were thinking about me. I think one of them found that encouraging and kept approaching me for that reason over the first week or two! But it was more in a hopeful nature than a teasing one, and he lost interest soon enough when I was clearly not that easy to get near.

I got over my self-conscious blushing issue soon enough and settled into my new environment comfortably. It was just different and strange, and it felt so nice to be popular for a change.

On the first day, as anticipated, Monique and Emma and the circle of girls that they were now friends with welcomed me with open arms. They were a calm, peaceful group of around eight or so girls, and I was surprised to find that pretty much all the girls in it were extremely kind—a rather rare thing in my experience so far!

The girls mostly sat around outside or at a table at recess and lunch time to talk hobbies and pleasantries, and I learnt quickly that a few of them had strong Christian backgrounds that made them very close. I wasn't religious myself, so it was cool that the girls were kind and tolerant of me regardless, and I never felt unwelcome on that basis.

But as time passed and my novelty wore off, I did start to notice myself slowly becoming restless within the group. At first, I couldn't understand why I felt so out of place there, as the girls really were lovely, and I puzzled to put my finger on where the discomfort was coming from. It's hard to describe exactly what it even was—a frustration, an itch to get more air time myself to talk about personal and deep things.

Perhaps the group was too large and the dynamics of the conversation were a bit paralyzing. In such a sizeable circle of smiles and chatter, I found myself a rather silent member of the group and somewhat frustrated with my inability to express myself. But I couldn't place or articulate those feelings. I didn't know about my Aspie self yet.

A few times, I tried to re-initiate going off and spending regular one-on-one time with Monique the way we used to back in the day. We did that a little, but she was no longer interested in spending all her time with me. She'd grown and moved on to wanting to talk about boys and center herself in the larger group. Gossip was the new and exciting social norm, and she had a talent for telling exciting stories and having the girls in stitches. I didn't understand why she'd changed and where my old best friend had gone.

And so the year went on, with me sort of lingering on the side of that group, fitting in but feeling out of place at the same time. Back in my class time, I took a lot longer to come out of my shell, as I didn't know anyone in my math and science electives, which were strongly predominated by males. All the girls in the group had chosen humanities or much simpler subjects, so it probably took me a good several months or so to really start talking to those classmates.

However, once I did break the ice with a few of the guys in my maths[16] classes, I realized a few things rapidly. For one, guys weren't as scary as I'd thought, and two, I clicked far better with the boys in my classes than I ever had with any girls. They were more consistent, straightforward creatures whose style of thinking was comfortable and familiar to me. Something just felt "right."

Within a few weeks into the term, a few of the more intelligent guys, whom I suppose may stereotypically have been described as "nerds," became my particular friends, and I started spending my lunchtimes with a group of six or seven guys instead of the girls. It was irregular, and I think at first, it caused some offense among the girls' group that I'd first spent my time with. They must have assumed I was ditching them for male

[16] Maths is my Aussie slang for Mathematics.

attention, and it was true that I seemed to get more attention from that group, but there was a lot more to it than that. I just felt at home in this group in a way that I hadn't before. Finally, a niche I could fit into.

Over time, I became more and more involved as a core part of the "guy group," as I would call it, and started spending time with them after school as well. They'd created a small garage-style band, and we would go to alternating people's houses for band practice every week or two.

I wasn't much of a musician myself, but I dabbled with playing chords on the guitar for the sake of being part of the group. To this day, I still only know how to play a few chords and not much more. I even attempted a little singing for one of the songs. The band wanted to take itself seriously and recruited a new young drummer who was quite talented. It never took off into much of anything, but we had a lot of fun.

We wandered the bushes near one or two of the guys' houses and played in old bush lands and a hidden overgrown amphitheater, talking about our music and random other teen chit-chat. At one of the guys' birthday parties, we had to dress up in 1940s outfits, and a small group of us went into McDonalds to get supplies. To my teenage mind, that was hilarious! I have so many memories of giggling and innocent mischief. It was the highlight of my high school years.

Back at school, I know there were some raised eyebrows at the fact that I was hanging on to this group of guys so closely, as I do like to make intimate friendships, and so I knew each guy well. Sometimes, I could be particularly chatty with two of my closest friends in the group, and I was told off in class more and more frequently for talking too much at the wrong moments! But at the same time, the teachers sort of had a soft spot for me as the good student, and I was never chastised too badly.

Come the end-of-year graduation celebration, I remember arriving in a fancy car that my guy friends and I had hired as a group. I dressed myself up in a long, blue, slimming dress and felt like the belle of the ball sitting at the guy table for the dinner portion of the event. Looking back, I still didn't know how to make myself up well— my eyebrows were too thick, and my face was plain. But I looked naturally pretty and slender and was feeling at home at my table with all my guy friends. It was a night to be excited about.

There was music and a dinner, and after a long evening of excitement, each of us was invited to come to the stage one by one to receive a token of our graduation. I can't recall now what we were handed. A certificate? A signed Bible? However, the thing that really did stick with me was the short speech I received when I walked up. A girl read out, with a tone of humor and light teasing, "Most girls have trouble finding one boyfriend in high school. Michelle has seven!"

And then, suddenly, I was walking up to the stage, a little taken aback, because you would think there could be other positive things that I could have been remembered for on that night. To imply I was having a relationship with all the guys was a little degrading for the importance of the moment, and I was a little tired of being misunderstood that way. But anyway, I'm sure it was all in fun, and I walked up and received my prize with a smile anyway.

I could complain about it, but then again, after high school, I did go on to date one of the boys from the group and ended up in a relationship with him for the next three years, so I guess I can't protest too loudly!

CHAPTER TEN

ASPERGER'S SYNDROME AND GENDER IDENTITY

So, as you may have inferred from my previous chapter and my experiences in high school, I've always been a little troubled by society's tendency to divide everybody into two distinct gender groups and automatically expect me to slot into "female world." For me, my *gender identity*—that is, how masculine or feminine a person feels on the inside—is ambiguous.

Yes, I'm physically and sexually female, and my body does come with that cocktail of unfortunate emotional hormones . . . you know what I'm referring to! But in many other regards—in the way I think, communicate, and relate to others, the way I approach tasks and make decisions, my logical outlook, and the way I like to joke and have fun—it's clear to me that my mind is really much more like that of a male, and it's frustrating that because I act and dress in a feminine way, people automatically want to lump me with the girls, where I don't feel comfortable.

Back in high school, I think I was fortunate to discover that I clicked so well with the type that we all know as the "nerdy guys." It gave me a place to fit in that I wouldn't otherwise have had and a chance to have those good intellectual and technical conversations that I sometimes craved. At that point in my development, it was something I needed.

At the time, the girls at my school were busy making small talk and chatting about interests I wasn't yet into. And they could get soooo tediously serious in their tone of conversation. So please don't hate me for saying this, but at the time, it just led me to conclude that women are really boring on the whole! Whereas when I would wander over to the boys, they were often engaging in lighthearted ribbing and banter that was fun.

There was a sort of freedom that came with the way guys speak without fear of offending. Guys tease because they like and respect each other, so little of it is ever taken to heart, unlike with women, who can be quite bothered by a stray social faux pas. For me, it gave me a social safety net, so I wonder why others found it such a shocking and socially inexplicable thing that I should want to be around guys in preference to girls.

Anyway, coming back to the present, you can imagine how amused I was a few years ago when I first discovered Simon Baron-Cohen's study on the extreme male brain theory of Autism. I didn't know whether to laugh, cry, or yell a big "I told you so" to all the people out there who insisted my wanting to hang with the boys was just out of place. It was validating in such a satisfying way.

For those of you who aren't familiar with the theory, it comes from a paper that first appeared in *Neurodevelopmental Disorders Magazine* in 1999. Simon Baron-Cohen presented a study in which he had devised a series of questions to determine male and female behavioral patterns. The idea was that males are stronger at "systemizing" behaviors and females "empathizing" behaviors (defined below). So one's gender could be determined by where a person sits on the systemizing-empathizing scale.

> **Systemizing** is defined as "the drive to analyze or construct systems" that "follow rules." It also involves being able to predict the behavior of a system (as opposed to predicting or understanding the behavior of other people). Males are, on average, more skilled at "systemizing" than females are. Think of mathematicians and engineers as good systemizers.

> **Empathizing** is defined as "the drive to identify another person's emotions and thoughts and to respond to these with appropriate emotion." It also involves being able to predict the behavior of people. Females are, on average, more skilled at "empathizing" than males are. Think of therapists and teachers as good empathizers.[17]

Interestingly, when Autistic people were tested, *both* sexes sat on average further toward the male (systemizing) side of the scale than typical males. Hence Baron-Cohen's inference that Autism may be a form of "extreme maleness of the brain."

---

[17] Foden, Teresa, et al., The "Extreme Male Brain": An Explanation for Autism?," IANCommunity (Interactive Autism Network Website), Feb 23 2010, http://www.iancommunity.org/cs/understanding_research/extreme_male_brain

So if you follow that logic the study implies, I should be somewhat like a girl but with a male-brain mode of thinking. Ha, what a surprise!

Now, I should note that this theory was never proven or accepted as fact. In fact, reading around on the topic, I've seen a lot of criticism about how systemizing and empathizing is far too narrow a criterion to measure people on, and the common consensus seems to be that Autism and Asperger's are a lot more complex than just extra "maleness." So I guess this theory should be taken with a grain of salt.

But just my own two cents: If someday this study was expanded to show "maleness" in a wider variety of behaviors (or brain scans), I wouldn't be arguing with the concept that my brain was more male than that of my peers. It explains my adolescence. And I wish more people would accept the concept that not everyone fits in the gender boxes a little more and get off my case, because it really has been a socially challenging thing!

Going out and about and trying to fit into female groups at school or in mums' groups, I've encountered a lot of negativity because of my "non-female" way of thinking. Women expect a lot from other women. They expect us to be nurturing, empathetic, and compassionate and display it in all the right ways.

They expect us to pick up on subtle cues and know what social and emotional responses are required and when. When to get up and help with something. When to ask another heartfelt question. When to give someone a hug. They expect us to know when a friend potentially might be upset or want to talk about something and prompt them to open up by asking the right warm and gentle questions. They expect us to remember all the social details of each other's lives—interesting and boring alike—and utilize them in conversation.

When a male makes a social blunder, he can be somewhat forgiven for being a "mere male" (which is misandry, I know). But if a female does it, it's as if she's committed an intentional act of harm, which is a severely offensive thing to do! Women will, of course, rarely tell you to your face what you've done wrong. They naturally expect that you know, even when you genuinely don't. And when other women look at me, they see female, so they expect all of this from me.

I can think of many times where I've been silently "dissed" by one female in my life or another and left to wonder what on Earth I might have done wrong. It can be confusing and seemingly out of the blue when I suddenly feel that subtle coldness or distance that wasn't there a minute ago. Over time, I've come to see that women like to always act sweet toward one another because it helps keep the peace. So when women do compete or "fight," it's usually passively, in a way that requires a high level of social savvy to follow. It is a complicated world that I can't always make out.

Living in my own little world, I personally don't react in those ways myself, and they're lost on me. Perhaps I don't have the perception skills to fully understand the messages being conveyed, but unfortunately, I've encountered them enough to make me wary of new women in my life—wary in the sense that I can like them but still fear they could suddenly dislike me or walk away from me tomorrow. Nowadays, I no longer just trust the words that people say. I need to take my time to look at people's actions to confirm if they're really sincere.

It's sad that I've come to feel this way, but I think it's a natural consequence of not reading people's feelings and motives well in a society that can be sometimes covert and unkind, especially to those who don't behave like the "norm." The good news, however, is that I'm forever learning and growing as I go, and the older I get, the more I do seem to fit in and transition more toward female acceptance. And as I do, I'm slowly learning to be more trusting again. Maybe one day, I'll even find myself fitting more with the women than the men. Who knows! It all seems to be a game of catch up.

But moving on . . .

Another major problem I've faced a little too frequently in my life is this idea society has about appropriate gender separation. If you fit in well with your own gender group, it may not be something you've ever noticed, but people do segregate the sexes naturally in many social environments. The girls move together to "talk," and the guys congregate elsewhere, such as around the barbeque. If it's just a casual social gathering, I usually buck the trend and go hang out with the guys anyway. Maybe this looks bad to the women. They assume it's sexual or predatory behavior, but it's just me moving to where I can feel comfortable.

And then there are times when there's enforced separation—you are a girl, so you must go to the girls' event. You are not welcome to join the guys. And this has become a major pet peeve.

I don't think anyone likes being excluded from their social groups for any reason, let alone for being the wrong gender. It's not something that I have control over, and it feels unfair. Yet it's something that I've experienced on several occasions. It serves as a harsh reminder that I'm not really a valid part of the only groups that I feel welcome in.

I remember there have been times when I felt hurt and discouraged that no one ever spoke up on my behalf and said, "Hey, don't cut Michelle out. She belongs here with us." But often, I guess people don't want to do that because it would seem out of place. Culture recognizes gender separation as a perfectly valid way to divide groups, and so I frequently found myself on the outside of what I thought was my own group. There's nothing I can do but accept it.

In early 2011, I remember having a moment where I was feeling particularly frustrated about which group in society I really fit into and wrote a post on Facebook on the topic of gender ambiguity. It read, "*I have concluded that I was born into a world of aliens. Men are from Mars, women are from Venus, and I'm not sure which planet I'm from but it is not one of these. I don't know why I was put in this world full of such strange creatures.*"

The thought first came from something my mother-in-law said to me many years ago. "Men are from Mars, women are from Venus, and Michelle is from Pluto." At the time, I thought she was insulting me. Maybe she was. But it was also quite perceptive of her.

Surprisingly, quite a few people "liked" the status, which I found interesting to note. It says to me that the feeling of "not fitting with the norm" resonates with many people—not just me—and probably for many different reasons. You would think that for a culture to become so strong in its views on roles and gender that most people would fit neatly into the round slots provided, but I think there are a lot of square pegs out there, wandering and looking for their place to be accepted too.

And when it comes down to it, I think it's a primal human need, to have a place where we're wanted and accepted by the people around us. To find a community that we fit into. Our peeps. Where we can sit without fear of exclusion or rejection for factors beyond our control. But, of course, in real life, that's so much easier said than done. Life is complicated. The world can unfortunately be a harsh place to live!

Though I should remember to be grateful that at least my mum let me be in that regard. Growing up, she allowed me a lot of freedom to explore who I was and hang out with whomever I saw fit, regardless of gender or the fact that I was often the only girl in the group. And thank heavens for that! I can only imagine how much worse my life could have been had I not been given that sort of leniency.

Chapter Eleven

AS on Fashion and Shopping

Now, after so much seriousness, I wanted to veer onto a much more lighthearted topic. So prepare yourself for an Aspie discussion on fashion! And in particular, women's fashion.

I'll start by saying that I have a complaint to make! Who on Earth designed the layout of women's clothes stores? And why, why, *why* are there so many types of items? Short-sleeve shirts, skirts, camisoles, miniskirts, blouses, shorts, three-quarter pants, T-shirts, Jeans, boob tubes,[18] long-sleeve shirts, jackets, scarves, sunglasses, sleeveless tops, dresses, handbags, half-length shoulder tops, etc., all mixed together in a messy sort of chaos. I can't make any sense of this layout system! How am I ever supposed to find the item that I've come in to buy when everything is so buried?

When I go out to the shops looking for a specific thing, I get so tired of having to dig through rack after rack to actually even find the light-grey, long-sleeved shirt with V-neck that I have written on my shopping list. I mean, the system is all good and well if you're a creative type of dresser who likes to mix and match and is spontaneously inspired by the fashions around them, but I don't even know what to do with some of these clothing pieces. I want to classify them as tops or bottoms, long sleeve or short

---

18 boob tube = tube top

sleeve, but how do I handle this three-quarter semi-see-through overshirt? Argh! I can't catalogue my wardrobe. Help!

Then, just to make it even worse, if I venture into the dark depths of the shops, I often find the sale racks—assortments of items supposedly categorized by size, but argh. In reality, bits have been thrown here, there, and everywhere. I finally find a top that I like in the size M rack, and curses—this one is an extra large! Who would be so cruel as to do this to me? Then, to top it all off, like icing on the cake, the entire store is garnished with accessories thrown in willy-nilly among the actual clothes and on the mannequins to spice up the look. Not in the accessories section where they belong! It's a nightmare! I give up.

Sometimes, when I look at these places, I think that these aren't really clothes shops at all. No, they're Venus flytraps designed to prey on women. The store lures their victims in with the sweet promise of sales and markdowns and an array of brand items assembled on the mannequins out the front. A woman may have only come look-ing for a shirt, but before she knows it, she's surrounded by the sweet "scent" of skirts and necklaces and a cute pair of heels to match. She buzzes around happily for an hour and leaves the shop with six unplanned items. The clothing immersion gives her a high.

The only problem with this for me, of course, is that I don't *like* shopping just for the sake of it, and I definitely don't want to spend that long doing it! I dislike the noise and the crowds and having to filter through countless items only to find that the spe-cific things I'm after aren't available. If the internet only had change rooms, I wouldn't even venture into these women's stores, but alas, they don't, so it's an unfortunate ne-cessity.

So when I do go into those dreaded shops, my aim is simple: get in, get the items I'm after, and get out as quickly as possible. And hopefully try to pick up as many things as I can at once so that I can minimize how often I have to do it again. I *am* a woman, true, but as an Aspie, I think I missed out on the "happy, joy, I love shopping" gene!

I've often thought before that if only I could lay out the clothes the way I wanted to, then this shopping process could be so much less painful, even possibly fun. I would throw out brands altogether and categorize everything by type and size.

The first store in a mall would contain only women's long-sleeved shirts sorted accurately by size and then style. When I came into the mall looking for a long-sleeved shirt, I could visit that store and only that store to see every long-sleeved shirt in my size that the mall had to offer laid out in front of me. I would try a few on, choose between them, and leave without ever needing to visit another store. They wouldn't even stock those silly items that don't fit into any particular category. Who wears them anyway?

Of course, in doing things my way, the shops would make far less profit and deter women from overspending. So it's not actually a viable option. But why let reality get in the way of my dream? I would be happy. I would take my new long-sleeved shirt home and place it in my long-sleeved-shirt pile in my similarly organized wardrobe right next to the short-sleeved-shirts pile and the full-length-trousers pile. Ah, the perfect wardrobe.

And odd as this may sound, it never occurred to me that my method of organizing clothes was unusual at all until I read an article one day referring to the way women like to lay things out. It seems these strange creatures (well, strange to me) organize by color or by brand, group matching outfits, or have no particular order at all in their wardrobes. They like it to feel a certain way or they want to have the flexibility to move things around to try out different mixes and matches. What an inefficient system. It no longer surprises me that some women take hours in the morning to get ready. I'm surprised such people can find anything at all!

So, as you may have guessed, I, like many Aspies, was not born with an interest in fashion and clothing, or at least it wasn't there when I was young. In my childhood and early teen years, I remember being teased occasionally on free dress days for wearing the odd daggy[19] thing my mum bought me. No one told me that you don't tuck your T-shirt into your jeans! What's wrong with black shoes and white trousers? Or the fluorescent-pink parachute tracksuit that my mum got me for my birthday?

In primary school, I recall wearing my school uniform one day on a free dress day because we'd been asked to pay a dollar for the privilege. I didn't care to dress up. The uniform was much easier, and I certainly didn't want to give up my dollar! I was so mad when they asked me to pay anyway.

But somewhere in my late teens, I did learn to take an interest in how to dress myself smartly. It wasn't because I suddenly fell in love with fashion so much as the sudden realization that the world treats you better when you present a smart and attractive image. It's sort of amazing when you discover just how obsessed with image the typical world is. It's like a powerful force.

It means having a much smoother time in both your personal life and the business world. It means being given what you want. It means interest from the opposite sex and getting away with things that you might otherwise not. It seems it's worth doing, and so, understanding that, I would be silly not to make the effort.

---

[19] A daggy person is someone who wears uncool stuff, most often overly casual gear such as T-shirts or tracksuit pants. Rather than an insult, it's often actually used as an endearing term to mean that you have no sense of style, but I like you anyway. A person who is a little clueless on modern trends might also be described to say daggy things, and I think the term dag historically referred to a bit of poo hanging off a sheep's bum. But I promise when we say it, we don't mean that anymore!

Nowadays, I do take pride in having nice clothes and looking attractive. In fact, I usually dress so well that it makes me look mistakably neurotypical and can easily confuse the people around me.

However, should you see me in a shopping mall, don't expect me to stop and make small talk with you. My smart, classy look may fool you, but I'm not there to socialize. I'm on an Aspie mission, scanning for items that meet the criteria I'm after. I probably won't see you there, let alone acknowledge you! Don't take it as rude. It's just the way I shop, battling the epidemic of the ever-expanding chaotic women's clothing stores! There's no time to acknowledge the existence of passersby. This is war! I'm on the hunt!

CHAPTER TWELVE

WHAT IS "WRONG" WITH ME?

Oh, wow. Have I got some news for you. Just two days ago, I did something brave. I let the cat out of the bag to my in-laws about my Asperger's Syndrome after all these years of them knowing me and not being aware of it.

Now, I can't say that I was brave enough to actually do it directly or attempt a verbal explanation and discussion with them. Oh no, doing it with words would have been far too scary for me. But this time, I had a large chunk of this book written, the backbone story of my life. So I printed it out—then forty pages—and handed it to my mother-in-law (with my fingers secretly shaking). She and my father-in-law were holidaying in Houston at the time and had been staying in a hotel nearby, allowing her to visit us frequently.

I told my mother-in-law to read the letter when I wasn't around. I said that I didn't want any detailed feedback and that I needed to finish this process on my own and from my own perspective, though, truth be told, I was probably more scared of negative feedback and perhaps afraid to see her reaction. So she took it away with her.

After handing it to her, the stress set in a little. It's hard to help doing that Aspie thing of playing a worry over and over in my mind, stressing about the outcomes. This is a big deal to me, after all, exposing myself to the people who form the permanent core of my life. (The boys and their grandparents have always remained close.) Will it be acceptance or rejection? I know it will have made my mother-in-law emotional.

She's the type who feels things deeply and would probably react a lot to each and every experience I shared.

I started going through possible ways she and my father-in-law could respond. Was I going to get a talk on how I was "viewing everything wrong" or how I "need to change X and just get in there and do Y and stop overthinking it"? I guess I expect these sorts of comments, because they're the usual reaction I get from people when I make little hints that something might be hard for me. People so often downplay my issues. "Everyone else deals with Z, so you should be fine dealing with Z too." "Nobody likes working, but we all do it." So that's what I waited to hear.

I thought about how one thing I particularly hate is the line "toughen up" or "harden up," which, fortunately, I haven't encountered excessively but have seen so often used on other people with little insight or real understanding. I wonder why the speaker assumes they know what that person is really going through to judge in this way. How could they possibly?

If the world's issues were as simple as changing a person's attitude, then counselors and psychiatrists would be out of business. Of course people don't just choose to be depressed, anxious, or whatever else they're dealing with. They're fighting against these things. And it bothers me that people retort like that, even in ignorance. It's one of the reasons that speaking up for people like me can be so confronting.

Another thing that went through my mind is how much I dislike it when adults take it upon themselves to coach me on "fixing" my behavior (when I really just came to them wanting someone to listen, not for help).

I had a lady do this to me once. She would describe to me how I was doing specific things wrong. I should change to become more like this instead; i.e., neurotypical. "Try doing this. Try saying that." More and more until my real self was almost unrecognizable. "That's better. You seem sort of neurotypical if you do it that way."—and completely unlike myself—"That's still not quite good enough, but it's an improvement. I'm telling you these things to help you fit in better." As if I haven't already changed more than a person should ever have to.

In my head, I get agitated when I hear talk like that, and I always want to reply, "Enough! I don't want to change any more. I've almost lost the real me in doing it, I'm bending over so far. I've spent so much time now trying to undo the damage that comes from self-denial and trying to be something that's not me, and I'm finally happy with the direction I'm finding.

"The last thing I need is people telling me I'm not good enough as I am and should bend over backward to fit into their stereotypes. What I really want now is to reverse the process. Let my quirks come out. My real self is fun and humorous and cheeky. Why should I shut that down? Why can't people learn to enjoy that little bit of randomness that is me? I think it's about time the world started to bend back a little and show some acceptance of who I am. I just want to be me."

But unfortunately, on the spot, I don't usually have the words to express these sorts of thoughts.

Anyway, when my father-in-law rang in the afternoon to say they would be coming around, it sounded a bit to me like, "Okay, I think we need to talk," (or that's how I interpreted it) and I braced myself for a potentially uncomfortable discussion.

As they headed over, I contemplated how I didn't want to engage and started to run through my side of the imaginary conversations in my head. "I don't want advice. I don't need to be helped. I'm fine the way I am. I don't need other people to try and 'motivate' me or push me to go for things. I already push myself hard enough . . ." But it turns out, I didn't need to say anything.

When my mother-in-law came over, she handed me a letter and said she thought she would respond like for like. And then they took Isaac (my older son) to the park and disappeared for a while to give me time to read. A letter! What a relief! All that stress and defensiveness for nothing.

Looking back, I wonder now why had I been so ready to argue? It's interesting that I made the automatic assumption that I need to debate to justify my views and people won't naturally respect my opinions and feelings. Being me and explaining myself has typically been so exasperating. Of all the responses I'd thought through, the one thing I hadn't predicted was for them to be accepting of what I'd written! Heavens. What was going on?

The letter read:

> Dear Michelle,
>
> Thank you for sharing your notes with me. I am pleased you trusted me with them. I loved your honesty. They explain clearly so many things to me, because, of course, like you, I have wondered over all these years why can't we talk/communicate more easily? What is wrong with me or her? To be honest, it is a relief to know what your condition is and that you are embracing it and in learning to understand it developing the positive side to Asperger's. I hope in the future you will teach me how to communicate with you in ways you find comfortable. [Some personal things.] Know that you all have our love and support.
>
> Celia

What a good reaction. What an unexpected reaction. Does that mean that I actually got through for once in a way that didn't just generate misunderstanding, judgment, and/or criticism? After all, helping others to understand what Asperger's really means was the whole point of the book. Could I actually be achieving what I aimed for here?

I was thinking, shortly after reading it, how happy I was to see the words "explained so clearly." I was understood! I'm actually starting to entertain the idea that I could be successful in my writing. What a great feeling! I'm motivated to write more. I want to change the world and alter society's view on Autism. I want people to "get it."

But enough getting carried away. While I'm talking about this letter, it raises another topic that I want to address, and please don't take it as me misinterpreting the letter. I understand that the letter was positive and kind and that my mother-in-law was being lovely about it all and I don't mistake the meaning. But it does raise the question of what is "wrong" with me.

If my mother-in-law views it that way, then I'm sure a lot of neurotypical readers will probably have similar reactions. I must have some failure or disability, right? I mean, that's why I was given the label "Asperger's" in the first place. The problems I am having have to be due to my own failings. My "condition." It's what is "wrong" with me.

What I really feel the need to say here is that there is *nothing* wrong with me. I'm just different. And any difficulties I have are the result of trying to live in a world where everyone around me is so different from me, not because I myself am faulty. I think Tony Attwood hit the nail on the head when he said, "People don't suffer from Asperger's Syndrome. They suffer from other people."

I'm not "wrong." I'm everything I'm supposed to be and more. But both the social world and the business world that I live in aren't set up for someone like me. I'm the proverbial square peg trying to fit in a round hole, and I can't function effectively like this. I have so much potential to be useful, creative, even ingenious. The world just has to find a way to utilize me better.

To come up with a rather bizarre analogy, as I often do—my mind is strange and visual—imagine taking a pack of dogs and adding one chimpanzee. Is the chimpanzee faulty because it's not acting like a dog? Is it a retarded dog or a dog with disabilities? No, it's just a chimpanzee. It isn't supposed to act like a dog. But if we leave the chimp in this situation indefinitely, it's going to have a pretty hard time living in a place where status is determined by the ferocity of one's bark.

I mean, it'll probably take on dog mannerisms and even learn to bark to fit in. It'll get better and better at this with time. But it'll always be a chimp, and it'll always stand out as different. But who's to say that being a dog is better than being a chimp anyway? The dogs are the majority, but that doesn't make them superior.

In a similar vein, who is to say that being "neurotypical" is superior to being an Aspie? Some people—Einstein, Isaac Newton, Bill Gates, and many other famous and/or highly successful people—are suspected to be Aspies. If you Google the topic of famous people with Asperger's, you'll see that the list is lengthy.

Heavens, I've even seen some people posting on Aspie forums how they think Asperger's is the next step in evolution. An advanced form of the human race. I wouldn't go as far as to say that, but I do think we're at least a side-step. And I wish people weren't so quick to assume we must be lesser.

To share a joke that I once found online, here is an article I once saw about Neurotypical Syndrome (paraphrased, as I couldn't find the original). And please don't take this to be offensive in any way. It isn't supposed to be a dig at typical people, just a document to highlight the point that if you look enough, you can find weaknesses in any group where there are clear differences between people.

Neurotypical Syndrome:

Neurotypical Syndrome is a neurological developmental disorder characterized by irrational behavior, extreme obsession with social conformity, and a strong intolerance to seemingly minor differences in other people. Neurotypicals often insist in following unproductive and sometimes even self-destructive behaviors and rituals and may passive-aggressively compete with others with whom they should be cooperating. Neurotypicals may find it difficult to be alone.

In the learning environment, people with Neurotypical Syndrome can display extreme deficiencies in logical thinking, concentration, and problem-solving ability. They often resort to wildly emotive and unsubstantiated analogies to prove a point, as opposed to being able to focus on factual evidence and logical discussion.

Neurotypicals may have difficulty with direct communication and are more likely than regular people to tell lies. Sadly, as many as 994 in 1000 people suffer from this condition.[20]

I guess as an Aspie, I found it a little comical. You see, it's all about perspective.

To tell a somewhat amusing story, I had an odd experience once where I got to see just how much people assume the label "Asperger's Syndrome" meant I must be somehow "a little defective." Shortly after receiving my diagnosis, I began to seek out Aspie meetup groups online in the hope of finding information and connection.

---

[20] Based on recent reviews of epidemiology, which estimate a prevalence of one to two cases per two thousand people for Autism and about six per one thousand for ASD. Newschaffer CJ, Croen LA, Daniels J et al. The epidemiology of Autism spectrum disorders [PDF]. *Annu Rev Public Health.* 2007,28:235–58. doi:10.1146/annurev.publhealth.28.021406.144007. PMID 17367287.

There weren't many adult groups around where I lived, but I did find and join one local group for parents of children and teens with Autism or Asperger's, and I decided to turn up to one of the events at a children's bouncing castle play area. I may have been the Aspie, but I brought Isaac, my older son, along to join in the play and socialize. I was noticeably pregnant with Trent, my second son, at the time.

During the group, I was asked at one point by a parent when I'd found out that my son had Autism, and I decided to reply directly that he didn't (at least to my knowledge) and that I was the one with Asperger's Syndrome. After all, I thought I might as well be honest with the group if I want to find understanding. It was the first time I'd ever walked into a group being "openly Aspie." The group hadn't picked it up at all before that point.

The ladies responded with fascination and asked a few questions, which I started to answer, but I was shortly interrupted by Isaac and had to go rescue him from some play equipment. When I came back, I recall that one of the ladies was talking about me. She was saying, "Isn't it amazing to see one of them with a husband and children? To know that they can have kids or that they could even want to get married and have children . . ." She continued speaking in front of me as if she didn't expect me to think much of it. It was the most bizarre experience of my life.

I thought to myself, "Um, hello! I'm standing right near you, and I can hear what you're saying."

"One of them?" All my life, I've been considered "normal" and have been expected to behave accordingly. I'm as intelligent and capable as the next person, and if that person is not extraordinary, probably more so. I've never been called a "one of them." What an odd thing to hear!

Of course Aspies want to be in relationships. I don't know one who doesn't, although some may be a little jaded from relationship failures. And yes, some of us do and some of us do not want children. Some of us even have them! I did, and I know a few other Aspies with children. We're not non-human!

I should probably stop to clarify that I wasn't angry from this encounter. I was just baffled by it. Is this what it feels like to be a labeled person? To be singled out as being different? It occurs to me that this isn't dissimilar to the feeling that a thin, attractive person might get when they dress in a fat suit to experiment with how differently the world treats them—the shock of experiencing being perceived as someone different and how it changes the way you're responded to.

Of course, no one was actually being mean to me in any way, and I'm not upset, but I definitely did get a feeling of being alienated and regarded as not one of them. What a bizarre feeling!

I guess this sort of response shows me the level of misunderstanding that there is out there in society. Perhaps this was a mum of a severely Autistic child. If that were so, then relationships and family may not be something that they can hold strong hopes for. But it still surprises me that people know about high-functioning Autism and Asperger's and yet they assume that there's still a giant unfillable gap between this and a "normal" person. And these are the parents, the ones who are supposed to be more educated on the syndrome.

I didn't go back to that group. It felt a little too odd and uncomfortable for me. Wouldn't you feel strange too if you were labelled as "one of them"?

CHAPTER THIRTEEN

UNIVERSITY

And now, back to the next installment of "the peculiar life of Michelle."

After graduating from senior school and thus having to leave my comfortable high school lifestyle, I decided to go on and take an engineering/science degree at university. It was actually a surprisingly simple thing for someone like me to organize. I applied—I can't remember now if it was by submitting a form or online— and then I got in. There was no interview or assessment of my suitability as a student, as my grades were high enough to fall into the automatic acceptance range. Just a letter in the mail saying congratulations for being accepted into the course and please come in on such-and-such date for orientation week. And so that's what I did.

I remember my mum questioning at the time if I really wanted to do such a long, technical degree or if something simpler and shorter would suit me better. But for me, it seemed the simple path to follow. I was good at maths, I was good at science, and there in the 1998 university course handbook I'd been given in school was a degree with both. I didn't really have any concept of what else was out there or any other way to go about it. I was rather oblivious to the world of other applied degrees and options that were available.

Settling in to university, I wish I could tell you stories of the wild parties or fun college experiences that I had, but actually, I was boring. I commuted in to university and back home for an hour by train every day and stuck mostly to what you would expect a nerd to do. I worked hard and didn't get involved in much extracurricular activity. (I lived so far away, it was hard to stay on campus that late anyway.) I focused on being on top of my workload and spent most of my free time working hard to get high marks.

Yeah, I was *that* person, the one who always had their head in the books, but with a bit of a crazy, playful personality unexpectedly thrown on top. One of my friends used to refer to me as "eccentric."

I know that for many Aspies, university (or college) is a time in which we struggle to cope and organize ourselves well enough to function, but for me, it was a place where I thrived. I mean, I, too, had the usual Aspie struggles—difficulty multitasking, poor natural executive functioning[21]—but I invented systems that worked for me and mastered them well.

My diary was my second brain and the center of my life! Any time any little thing came up that I would need to remember later, out it would come. I wrote daily lists of things I had to do, and each morning, I would go through the list and prioritize the work for the next few days. It was something I actually looked forward to doing, and sometimes I would even reprioritize my lists multiple times a day just for fun—yeah, I know I'm weird!

I must have been visibly obsessed with it too, as I remember one guy in my class, Chris, having some fun one day. When I opened up my diary one morning, there in the task list, a new item had been added: "Shag Chris." I'm pretty sure I didn't write that myself!

When it came to working and trying to socialize at the same time, I quickly learnt that that was just not going to happen. I don't have that multitasking brain that most of you are lucky enough to be born with, so for me, it was either "work mode" or "social mode" only. Thus, I simply decided: socialize at university, work at home. No stress, no guilt—it was my system. With people constantly talking to me and making noises around me at university, it was either that or frown and shush people all day! So I opted for the more polite route.

Of course, that made me rather relaxed at university, and I think sometimes in class, I may have annoyed people by talking a little too much. I made sure I always wrote down the material so I could study it later, but generally, I wasn't always paying

---

[21] In case you're unfamiliar with the term, "Executive function and self-regulation skills are the mental processes that enable us to plan, focus attention, remember instructions, and juggle multiple tasks successfully. Just as an air traffic control system at a busy airport safely manages the arrivals and departures of many aircraft on multiple runways, the brain needs this skillset to filter distractions, prioritize tasks, set and achieve goals, and control impulses." Harvard University, Centre on the Developing child, http://developingchild.harvard.edu/science/key-concepts/executive-function/

that much attention, and I've never been great with volume control. My friend, Chris, once asked if perhaps I might be partially deaf because of my tendency to talk too loudly or quietly for no reason, though it turns out I'm not.

I recall one particularly embarrassing day when I was having a more personal chat with a friend and had one of those moments where the room suddenly went quiet, leaving me saying loudly to the whole room, "Yeah I have pretty small boobs." Hopefully one day, I'll live that down!

The downside of my all-work-or-all-play system, of course, was that once I got home, I had a huge amount of extra work to do, and I spent most of my weekends sitting on my bedroom floor with my head buried in books and paperwork.

The lectures were often hard for me to grasp when I was in class—I only seem to catch every second sentence from verbal communication—so for every hour I spent in a lecture, I think I spent about two at home, re-reading the notes and learning the material. It made weekends quite a drag, so, contrary to most people, I used to look forward to my Mondays coming around when I would be free to play and chatter again.

I don't think I ever had any spare time on weeknights or weekends, given my constant workload, but I did take a lot of solace in being alone in my room or the lounge room being able to look at the weird array of flowering cherries, conifers, rhododendrons, maples, etc., that made up my mum's concept of gardening. We had six and a half acres of land with a small creek at the back, and Mum had a passion for planting garden beds. In some parts of the house, the trees from the porch stretched over toward the trees in the garden and almost made little arches of flowers at the right time of year, like a little fairy garden. I loved walking through that area.

When I needed to wind down, I would often put on my gum boots[22] and walk down into the yard just out of the view of the house. I would sit on a fallen tree and enjoy the peace that came with being able to look 360 degrees without a house or person in sight. It was my calming place. (Although I did have to watch out for the leeches!)

Back at university, I found my first year socially challenging. The sizes of the first-year classes I was in—chemistry, math, and biology—were colossal (maybe a thousand students over three streams of a subject), and it took a long time for me to be thrown together with the same people long enough to befriend anyone.

But by the third year, I was able to settle into a much smaller engineering group—mostly guys—and became familiar with the people who frequented the chemical engineering common room. I was comfortable there and enjoyed my little common room niche, and it made me a lot happier to have a place like that to base myself.

In those later years, I had a few particular friends. I became good friends with one guy, Chris (the "shag Chris" guy), at the start of second year university when he

---

[22] Gum boots = Tall, waterproof rubber boots, commonly worn in Australia, also known as galoshes.

first transferred in. He would sit next to me in all my classes, and people would tell me he was frequently in the common room looking for me. I have to say it was a bit of attention I very much enjoyed. As I got to know him, it unraveled that he was quite troubled, but I have to say his complexity made him one of the most interesting people I've ever met. Sometimes, people—even though troubled—can be a deep and satisfying addition to your friendship circles.

Another guy in the class, Alex, sticks in my mind because he used to talk and play silly games with me during the lectures, such as rubbing out what I was writing while I was writing it down. He even once cut off a little piece of my hair! Sometimes he drove me crazy, but I forgive him that. He was a good guy overall. Perhaps an unusual one, but he turned out to be quite loyal as a friend.

And, of course, there were Colin and Sam, whom I worked with on a major project in final year. Sam invited me over to her house for small social gatherings and was always stable and supportive. Colin loved to gossip, and the two of us spent vast amounts of time together and had some great humorous, mischievous conversations.

Sometimes, my life was so unique in funny little ways that as we were walking around, Colin would make jokes about us being on *The Michelle Show*; i.e., where there were hidden cameras filming our every move. At the end of the year, Colin submitted a passage about me to the annual magazine, which read, "Sadly, there is not enough room on the rogue sheets to include for Michelle. This is a crime, since Michelle has had so many embarrassing moments, from those outbursts in lectures to those discussions with Alex. In reality, we could devote a whole magazine just to Michelle, and perhaps someday, someone will."

And ironically, someone did end up writing about me one day—forget a magazine. It was a whole book! But I never realized that that person was going to be me!

Socially, I would say those university days were some of the happiest times of my life. The oddities of academia made me a good fit with those around me, all of whom I would still consider to be good friends if I had much contact with them now. But as time went on, unfortunately, most of us moved away to one location or another for work reasons. Long-distance friendships tend to slip away over time.

My later years at university were also the time when I met Robert, whom I would eventually go on to marry. He was taking chemical engineering also and graduated a year ahead of me, although I didn't get to know him well until the end of his graduation year. Just as the year came to a close, he invited me to join him at a final year celebration being held by a group of students that weren't going to the official Chem Eng ball.

I remember he picked me up in what he and his brothers called "the truck," an older, red vehicle with no roof. We had a lot of fun cruising around town there and back with the wind blowing through the car, and Robert and I got to really talking for the first time. He was deeper than I'd realized and had a subtle and dry sense of humor—an educated wit that I quite liked. He was also young and innocent and a kind, gentle sort of person. You could just sense that about him. By the end of the night, I declared him "good company," and we made plans to hang out again. Things took off from there.

I remember Robert enjoyed building on Colin's jokes about *The Michelle Show*, and when we would go on dates, he would point out a rainbow and tell me he ordered it in especially for me. His lines were mostly cheesy and sometimes taken from movies, but it moved me. He was trying. And so, we continued to see each other on weekends through the next year while he took a job at a site a few hours away, and I plugged away at my final year of engineering and science studies.

As I continued on with the final subjects in my degree, I discovered that my chemical engineering coursework wasn't turning out as interesting as I had first hoped it would be. I guess I chose the course because I thought engineering would be a good field to get work in and I wouldn't have to write or deal with people too much. Ha! Well, that worked out to be a bit of a joke, and in reality, it was work that forced me to develop a lot more social and writing skills.

A few of my subjects were more systematic and very "me" (I loved Chemical Process Analysis), but many were ho-hum, and my passion wasn't strong. I wish I'd pursued genetics, ecology, psychology, statistics, algebra, or one of the areas I was passionate about. But at the time, I was pressured to do chemistry and only the subjects I could fit in alongside my engineering degree, so unfortunately, I dropped the things that fascinated me the most.

I think that back then, my understanding of the purpose of university was solely to set yourself up to get a "good job," "good" meaning solid pay and lots of employment opportunities available. I never questioned that idea or thought about the concept of learning for enjoyment until much later.

I wish someone had pointed out to me then that I was going to be working for the rest of my life and that I should do something that I love. And that if you're passionate enough about it, the jobs will follow. I wish I'd understood that there's so much more to life than working and earning money. Money is a means to an end, not "who you are." Finding a life that makes you happy should be the real goal. To follow one's passion is a beautiful thing, and I was strongly passionate about a few things. But instead, I made logical choices that led me away from them. We live and learn.

Regardless, I was motivated to succeed, and succeed I did. I graduated university with an average grade of 85, placing me somewhere near third when compared to those I studied engineering with (the class that graduated one year before me), in a class of around 100. I was extremely capable of achieving the goals I put my mind to, and university taught me to have a lot of confidence in myself and my abilities. I used to picture myself flying—soaring across the top of the world. I was headed up and up. Just imagine what I could've done if I'd pursued real areas of interest!

Unfortunately, this was probably the peak of my success, and after graduation, I ran into the business world, which wasn't the devil I knew. It turned out to be a world that I didn't have the skills to thrive in the same way, and I was in for a big shock. But anyway, we'll save that for the next story topic.

Chapter Fourteen

Asperger's and Memory

Q: I've heard some Aspies have an amazing ability to recall countless facts and data on their topic of interest. So tell us about your Aspie super-memory!

Oh, I wish. I wish I could sit here and start this chapter with a paragraph about rote memory, telling you just how brilliant mine is and recounting story after story about just how marvelous and talented I am. "I'm so good. I'm so good." But alas, it seems I'm actually no good at that at all.

Of all the cool Aspie traits to miss out on, it turns out that this was the biggest one I skipped. I know. It's so unfair! So, unfortunately, there will be no super-memory stories from me.

But while we're on the topic of Aspie memory, there's one other issue I would like to bring up, because I relate to this one in spades, and that is the ability to take in verbal instructions and the most simple day-to-day information.

Have you ever noticed how flaky we Aspies can be in this regard? You tell us about your pet dog's grooming difficulties and your second aunt's first and middle name and instruct us to wash the dishes and mow the lawn in one conversation. Then, the next day, it seems we've forgotten all the personal details and only done half the jobs we were asked. On the surface, it looks like such contradiction that we can be so strong at reciting useless (or even sometimes useful) facts on our favorite topic of interest and yet unable to recount the simple stuff.

But the reason this happens, I've learnt, is because the latter is not actually a memory problem at all. It's about us having difficulty *taking in* information in the first place. Sometimes, we just can't function with so much sensory and verbal input and real-time speed. Or if the topic is not of interest, it may be hard for us to keep our focus on it in the face of other input.

And I particularly wanted to bring it up in this chapter, because, for such a long time, I really thought it was some sort of memory glitch that I had, and I used to kick myself for how bad I was at grasping and remembering the little details that people would tell me about themselves. I must be selfish, right? To never be able to remember the details of other people's lives? Everyone else cares enough about other people to remember that stuff. What was wrong with me? It took me a long time to figure that one out—and a lot of guilt, I might add.

So, when does this so-called memory issue affect me? Well, unfortunately, I can be pretty bad with directions. For example, if you were to direct me by saying, "Go halfway down the street to the light and turn left. Follow the road almost to the end and turn right at the petrol station.[23] Take the first left immediately after and then left again into Whatsitsname Boulevard. We're house number twenty-three on the left with the blue letterbox," you know you're going to find me pulled over on the street to the left of that first set of lights! I can't remember any more words than that!

But the bigger difficulty that arises from it, I think, is just being able to recount all the things that happen in day-to-day social interactions. I don't know how many times I've found myself thinking back to a fast-paced conversation with friends and wanting badly to recall something that I remember came up and coming up completely blank.

"What was that 'play space' again that so-and-so was telling me about? Something about kids and pools and horses? Now would be a great time to take the kids to that . . . Argh, where was it? Who was it that I was talking to again?" Yet all I can bring up is some blurry image of horses in water that I only vaguely noted at the time.

I think a great solution for me would be if I could carry around a personal voice recorder to take things down as people spoke to me; e.g., "Jenny—new person, messy red hair; Aunt Susie May sick, liver edema, something about diuretics; two kids; dog with long coat, needs regular grooming; bakes raspberry muffins. Alice—pool almost finished, had a foot callus treatment, Sophie (daughter) refusing to go down at sleep time. Kids' play space 'Old McDonalds Farm' off the 59 freeway NE, FM 1960. Sounds great!"

---

[23] Gas station. In Australia we call gas "petrol."

But I think people would give me odd looks if I made a habit of recording their conversations! Heck, I already get some odd looks when I get out my diary to write down important facts from time to time. But it's my second brain, and I need it!

Sometimes, I like to consider myself analogous to an oddly designed computer, one that was built with a fantastic high-speed CPU but unfortunately low RAM. I need that pen and paper to act as an additional RAM module and temporarily store the data so that I can function to my true ability. Without it, all you'll see is that annoying "processing, processing, processing . . ." symbol.

So if you want to give me lines of instructions, seriously, let me write it down. It's not a sign of disrespect or lack of intelligence, just a lag in my ability to convert and memorize too many verbal instructions at once. And when given the right tools to take notes and store information, you'll find I'm a real nifty little machine!

CHAPTER FIFTEEN

SENSORY OVERSTIMULATION

Q: I've heard that some people with Asperger's can suffer from sensory over-stimulation. Do you experience this yourself?

Why, yes I do. End of chapter.

Just kidding, of course. You know you wouldn't get me to stop talking that easily!

Sensory overstimulation is definitely an issue I experience, like many of my Aspie peers, and it's an Autism symptom that, I have to say, I've always found baffling. I mean, Asperger's and Autism are all about social and communication differences and difficulties, and yet there, smack bang in the middle of the lists of traits, are light, touch, sound, taste, and smell sensitivities. How is that even linked to the same area of the brain, I've wondered. And also, why poor motor skills?

But regardless of the strangeness of the symptom, it seems that sensory hyper-sensitivity in people on the spectrum is a real and serious thing. For me, it's noise and light that particularly grate on my nerves. Oh, if only I could turn the volume down on people! Where is that switch? Don't people realize how loud their voices are? And who made the sun so bright? But these things are what they are, so we deal with it the best we can.

I read an article on this topic quite recently, actually, which I found rather fascinating. It was a new study pinpointing additional brain synapses as a possible underlying cause of Autism[24]—i.e., too much information is being passed from neuron to neuron within the brain—which could certainly shed some light on this link that's been puzzling me. How amusing it would be if such a complex condition as Autism could all be linked in the end to something as simple as excessive local brain signals. That would certainly make it easier to diagnose and work with.

But these are new hypotheses yet to be proven and reproduced, and I'm no expert on the matter, so whatever the cause, I'll move on to answering this chapter's question by discussing the areas I know about—the two great sensitivities that affect my day-to-day life: noise and light, and I'll also make a few comments on touch.

1. Light sensitivity:

It wasn't until diagnosis—much later in my adult life—that I actually realized I had light sensitivity, and quite badly at that! The signs were there, but it took me a while to put two and two together.

I knew I got frequent eyestrain headaches. I knew that I needed the brightness on my TV or computer fully down or it would hurt my eyes. I knew my mum or husband would sometimes tell me to stop frowning when I really wasn't, and sometimes, I couldn't stop. And then one day, it dawned on me: I'm not frowning. I'm squinting. In fact, I've spent so much of life squinting that I have a pronounced frown wrinkle between my brows, one of the only wrinkles that I have!

There were also other tells. I've always had dilated pupils, which I'm guessing might be linked, as I've met other Aspies who are the same way. In fact, I had one friend who said when he spaced out—daydreaming—sometimes people would think he was stoned. His pupils were always so large, they always looked dilated, which caused him the occasional problem! But the strongest giveaway, the one you think I would've picked it up from, is the way I feel when I'm in the sunlight.

How many times have people said to me, "It's a beautiful sunny day," or, "I hope the sun will be out tomorrow," and I've privately thought, "I really hope not! I hope for a pleasant, overcast day. Please give me miserable weather! The kind that makes me relax and feel at peace." I know that other people love frolicking out in the sun and enjoying the brightness of summer, but for me, having that direct sun on me drains my energy and has always made me, subconsciously, that little bit tenser. And no, before you suggest it, sunglasses don't fix it! They help, but they nowhere near solve the problem!

Sometimes, I've found the sunlight a big challenge when taking my children out to playgroups at parks. People just love to gather at parks, so there are often meetups there

---

[24] Belluck, Pam, "Study Finds That Brains With Autism Fail to Trim Synapses as They Develop," The New York Times (online), August 21 2014, http://www.nytimes.com/2014/08/22/health/brains-of-autistic-children-have-too-many-synapses-study-suggests.html? r=0

when the weather is "nice," and it's great for the kids. It's just unfortunate that I have to socialize in a setting with the added burden of the sun taking away the energy I need to make that extra social effort. Why can't we meet in some creepy, dark, shadowy place? That would be fun too, wouldn't it? A perfect place to bring little children. Do you think I could convince people? Oh well, I guess not.

In my last job, I remember how something amusing used to occur repeatedly. My boss, Tony, and I (both of us!) had a habit of arriving early in the mornings and sitting in the office with the lights turned off. He was a little light sensitive too, I believe, and it really wasn't that dark in the office with the sun rising outside, just pleasantly dim.

However, when other people arrived, we would constantly be asked, "Why are you two sitting in the dark?" And then they would disturb our peace by turning on all the lights. Flick, flick, flick. And in that instant, the fluorescent glare would be on me, and my restfulness would be gone. I hate that feeling of people flicking the lights on.

Tony and I continued the trend, and people continued to think it was strange. But I love the feel of a dimly lit room, and I had no intentions of changing that when I didn't have to. If I could have left the lights off all day, if other people had never come in, perhaps the office would have been a more pleasant place to be!

Sometimes in the evenings, I like to go for walks once the sun has started to set, and I enjoy that feeling of peace and darkness. It gives me a natural high. I'm alive again, like all the burden of the daytime has been lifted off my shoulders. It gives me the urge to skip down the streets and spin and twirl, absorbing all the life around me. That feeling is elation, and it's one of the few times I feel like I really know myself.

2. Sensitivity to touch:

Now, touch sensitivity is a topic I decided to slot in here at the last minute. I know it's a bit random, considering that I'm not someone who suffers a lot from touch sensitivity! I'm fine with various clothing fabrics and clothing tags, and touching odd textures doesn't irritate me, so I can't really relate to the extreme texture issues that some Aspies experience. However, I've noted a few things about myself in regard to physical touch that are sort of interesting.

I know that when I was young, I was always acutely aware of the sensation of someone touching me. At school, when people would brush my skin or touch my neck, it always felt uncomfortable or even a little alarming to me. I remember one day in high school how some girls started touching me on the neck repeatedly because they were amused at how I tensed up and reacted. It became a joke for them to try and get that reaction out of me.

I do remember that as a child, my mother almost never hugged me, and for most of my life, I assumed that this was because she wasn't the physically affectionate type or didn't wish to touch me. I found it sad and took it an indicator of a lack of affection for me. But in a recent conversation with her, she told me that as a child, I didn't like to be touched. I withdrew. She said I pushed away her attempts to hug me, so she stopped trying. So it seems that maybe I started it!

Nowadays, as an adult, I wouldn't describe myself as particularly averse to being touched. From a partner, I enjoy general physical contact as a sign of shared affection. Similarly, with my own children, it feels natural, and I can enjoy it from people I have an intimate level of friendship with.

However, there's some degree of discomfort and awkwardness when less-familiar people try and hug or put their hands on me. I still tense up in the same way that I did as a child and secretly want to pull away. I always assumed that this was because I'm not used to it and I'm unsure of the proper way to react. There's a degree of self-consciousness that comes with it, and heaven forbid I put my boobs on a person the wrong way and give mixed messages! But who knows? I guess it does create a lot of feeling, which is sort of unwelcome from anyone but those who are closest to me. Is that supposed to be a part of the same sensitivity? I'm not sure.

3. Sensitivity to noise:

Last but not least, we come to noise, one of the most difficult sensitivities to avoid. Loud noises can be quite a problem for sound-sensitive oddities like me, because almost everywhere you go where there are people, there's going to be noise. And no amount of standing at the back or making grumpy faces at the crowd is going to solve that! (And no, I don't stand there doing that . . . well, much.)

When I was younger, I must've had a better ability to just tune the noise out and get along with my day despite the irritation, because I always could push through it. But nowadays, I find I can tolerate it less and less, perhaps due to having to deal with it for so long each day. I have friends on the spectrum who describe noises as being physically painful for them. One person I know, David N., likened it to someone stabbing him in the ear repeatedly. I never thought I had it that badly, but I have to admit, lately, with children in tow, it's starting to feel that way for me too.

It seems that for each Aspie, noise sensitivity can present itself differently in regard to which particular noises will set them off. Some people can't stand dogs barking. Meh, they're okay to me. And I can tune out kids playing better than most! But I do seem to have a lot of issues related to adults talking too loudly or too many adults talking at once.

For example, I find sports commentary irksome, especially as the commentator gets excited over the action unfolding and starts to raise his pitch . . . and he passes to so-and-so, and so-and-so passes to so-and-so . . . SO-AND-SO KICKS IT DOWN

THE LINE, AND IT'S A GOAL! [YELL A LOT MORE DETAILS HERE!]
Please don't put me in a car with someone who "just wants to catch the score" on the radio. I think I'd rather jump out the window while the car was going than suffer the drive! I won't look kindly at you turning the radio on.

Sometimes, it's just that person in the group with the unusually piercing forms of expression—you know, the one with the loud outbursts—who's too much to handle. My mother-in-law has a sudden, loud (hammering the eardrums) laugh. And I'm sorry, Celia, to put that in here. I still love you!

Another common sound barrier that I keep running into is that racket you get from large crowds of people, such as the type you find in a crowded restaurant or at a street gathering or festival. Of course, it's overstimulating and wears me down rapidly, as you would expect, but even more awkward than that, I seem to become socially inept in the noise and can't make out what anybody is saying!

I don't know how many times I've sat in a restaurant with friends feeling self-conscious because I just can't hear what the smiling face next to me is chatting away about. There are only so many times you can say "pardon" and "no" and "I agree"! I have no choice in the end but to fade out and stop trying to pretend. I've often had the feeling that I've become a third wheel, even when I'm sitting right in the middle of the group. It makes me feel really alone, as odd as that sounds.

For much of my teenage years, I suspected that perhaps I had problematic hearing because of how much difficulty I've had interacting with people and following what was going on when I get stuck in groups like this. However, in a visit to an ear doctor a few years back, I learnt that the opposite was true. The specialist told me that I would be the sort of person that would notice obscure notes in a symphony that (and I quote him) "us mere mortals wouldn't." My hearing was exceptional. So I asked him why I have so much difficulty understanding people, and he explained that it's a brain thing.

Who knew? It turns out my brain is different!

In fact, I learnt something interesting recently that suddenly made a lot of sense. Apparently, it's normal for human brains to be wired to tune in specifically to conversation over the background noise and chatter, so most people can communicate with each other more easily, even amongst a crowd. However, for some Aspies like myself, the brain doesn't differentiate the voice of the person talking to me over every other tap and click and conversation going on in the room.

So I've learnt that is my problem. I hear too well! I hear everything in the room simultaneously—every sentence, every person shuffling in their seat, every tap of a spoon or fork or dish, the song and any background buzz from the radio (I hate white noise), every single conversation going on in the room. No wonder I've been having all this trouble!

On a somewhat related note, talking on the telephone is another task I've always struggled with for reasons I can't quite pinpoint, although I'm pretty sure it, too, has something to do with my difficulties hearing what the other person is saying over the background static and making out their meaning without being able to watch for gestures or expressions on their face. I can do it well enough when I try, but it requires so much concentration to understand what the other person is saying back to me that it exhausts me. So it's a task I tend to avoid except for the people in my life that I'm most comfortable with—and unafraid to offend!

Socially, this can be a big setback, because so much catching up is done over the phone, and if you don't call people, they might make the assumption you're not interested in making an effort in the friendship. I get the impression with my mother-in-law sometimes that this is a barrier to our relationship. I think she leaves me alone because I don't contact her much, and maybe she sees me as aloof or disinterested in being close with the family. What she doesn't realize is that I don't call anyone.

In fact, the only people I've called voluntarily in many years are my mum and my partners. Then, much more recently, I also started to make the occasional call to my friend, Paula, whom I've started to get along well with and feel a certain degree of safety around. This is a *huge* breakthrough to me, to reach phone call level with a friend. It means I trust them so much that I'm not even afraid to lose them by misunderstanding and saying wrong things on the phone. It's almost unheard of for me to do it voluntarily. Yet I'm pretty sure Paula wouldn't even know it's a big deal. It's just something I started doing one day after many months of friendship.

Anyway, last but not least, I thought I would end my "noisy" section with a story about action movies, because the sound that action movies make when playing in the background is definitely a noise to top them all! They don't just sound like screaming and destruction. They're the sounds of screaming and destruction blasted right into my ears!

My little story is about one holiday when Robert (my husband at the time) and I had rented a house in Bright with two other couples who are close friends. I was heavily pregnant at the time with Isaac, so the other couples were quite accommodating and gave us the biggest room with an en suite[25] right up at the front of the house. It was actually a rather comfortable holiday where we all had fun sitting around the fireplace and even played games in our pajamas one evening, you know, just to embrace the stereotype.

Anyway, one evening, the boys decided that they wanted to sit in the main room and watch an action movie together in the evening. And that was fine. I wasn't par-

---

[25] A private bathroom adjoining a bedroom.

ticularly interested, so I excused myself and headed to bed, as I was awfully tired in my third trimester.

The problem was, however, that our room was the one in the house adjoining the main TV lounge area, and the sounds from the movie in the next room were loud. I lay in bed and tried to rest, but the noise was hurting my ears that little bit too much for me to sleep. It wasn't unreasonably loud for a movie viewing, just loud enough for the sudden loud bursts to grate.

I considered asking the boys to turn it down, but I couldn't decide if that was a reasonable and "normal" thing to do. You see, back at that point in my life, I was still very self-conscious and unaware of my different sensitivities. I spent a lot of time analyzing my actions to make sure my behavior was "right," and if unsure, I tended to err on the side of caution. I was unsure.

In the end, I was too agitated by it to stay in bed, so I went into the en suite, where the noises were quieter, shut the door, and made myself a little nest of towels on the floor to lay in. It was quieter, and at least I could get peace that way, though it was a little uncomfortable, and I awkwardly tried to rest. After around an hour, the noises *finally* stopped, and I was able to go back to bed and get some proper sleep.

These four people are among my best friends in the world and would probably be more understanding than anyone, but I guess this is what happens when you have no label to explain why your needs are different from others'. Repeat bad reactions to my seemingly fussy requests, which were actually quite serious for me, taught me not to ask for these "silly little allowances" any more. The world had me convinced that I was the one being fussy and unreasonable.

I've heard other Aspies say before that they would never wish it upon anyone to go through life with this syndrome not knowing what it is. And it's for reasons like this that I wholeheartedly agree. My life would have been so different if I'd only known then the things that I know now and been able to explain my needs better. It would have given me the confidence to actually ask for what I needed when I was uncomfortable. Imagine how much better my world could have been if I had only had that.

CHAPTER SIXTEEN

MY FIRST FULL-TIME JOB, WORLEY

"So, what happened? What went wrong when you entered the workforce?" you might ask. And isn't that the million-dollar question? Even with the blessing of hindsight and an understanding of my Asperger's, I still find it hard to describe exactly what the feeling was that I experienced when put behind a desk. But whatever it was, it was very wrong.

I think the crux of it was that suddenly, I wasn't able to do things my way any longer. I couldn't come and go as I pleased, I wasn't in control of managing my own time, and when I really just needed to walk away, there was no avenue for me to escape. All the systems and methods I'd come up with for coping with life's frustrations that had worked in the freedom of a study environment weren't accessible to me here. Socialize at work and get the work done at home? Not an option. Yet the mental exhaustion of trying to do both is insufferable to me! Too bad, suck it up. From 9 a.m. to 5 p.m., I was trapped.

And so, those five years that I worked, I fell into the heaviest depression I've ever encountered, which could have easily killed my spirit irreparably had I never found a way to get out. And the obvious question here is, why didn't I just stop? You think I would have just refused and walked away from it so many years earlier. Believe me, I wanted to, but socially, it was hard.

How do you explain to the people around you that what you need now is to just crash and do nothing for a while until your head feels normal again, when you don't even know what's wrong yourself? It always felt like a depression of completely unknown origin that I couldn't make sense of myself, let alone justify to others. "Think positive," people tell you, "and you can pull yourself out of it with an upbeat attitude." I worked so hard to fight it.

I remember when I first went in for my formal Asperger's diagnosis a year and a half ago now. Dr. Loveland, who diagnosed me, explained that these workplace experiences I describe weren't uncommon for people with Asperger's and that she'd heard stories like mine before. She explained to me that that "sick" feeling I talked of was the result of bottling up frustration and anxiety all day, every day. Built up over time, I suppose it manifests physiologically, causing me stomach upset, low weight, and a general feeling of being unwell.

Some others with Asperger's are known to have "outbursts," where the frustrations get too much and they yell or snap at those around them. Many Aspies have trouble holding jobs for that reason. I can't decide which is better: suppress it and feel unwell or act out and lose jobs. If you act out, I guess at least it's out of your system and you don't have to feel the way I felt. I don't ever want to feel those feelings again.

But back to the beginning . . .

At the time when I graduated university, the economy was at a slow point, and graduate jobs were scarce. Robert, whom I was soon to marry, had graduated the year before me and had gone to work in Sale, a town a two-hour drive from the city, so I was looking for a job that would allow me to see him. The options were a little limited. In fact, pre-graduation, I was only able to find two local chemical engineering roles to apply for.

One of these companies was Worley, a consulting company that, among other things, provided engineering services to the oil and gas industry. Worley had jobs in several "site" facilities (including Sale) as well as their main city office, so I thought they'd be an ideal place to apply.

When I went in for the interview, I immediately had a gut feeling that I wouldn't like the city office environment much. Something about the cubicle setup, the lights, the noise, the crowds, the lack of privacy or sanctuary . . . But, being one who suffers from social anxiety,[26] I put any negative feelings I had at the time down to that. I smiled, put on my confident act, and set about making a good impression at the interview.

---

[26] I talk a little later about social anxiety and how it relates to my Asperger's. But for those who are unfamiliar with the term, social anxiety is basically anxiety triggered by interacting with other people and is often linked to fears that others might think poorly of you. For some people, social anxiety can be so bad, they struggle to even act normally in the presence of other people and can freeze, have panic attacks, sweat, or have difficulty talking, making those fears well founded! Fortunately for me, my anxiety was never as severe as that!

Two interviews later, after receiving a lot of positive feedback, it had been established that there were no site roles available, and I was offered a job as a process engineer in the city office. I remember that moment quite well even now, all these years later. One of the interviewers said, "Congratulations," and we all smiled. But my smile was an act. Inside, I had a sinking feeling that was completely foreign and unexplainable to me. We shook hands and exchanged pleasantries, and I said I would get back to them soon. And then I went home.

The job seemed a good one. The role was solid and on a promising career track. It was a foot in the door to the process engineering world. The company had a pleasant culture, and it was the only such offer I was likely to get before graduating. I rang back the next day and told them how happy I would be to take the job.

Once working, I certainly didn't hate everything about the job. There were a few key tasks that really suited me, and being a process engineer was quite a good fit. I made HYSYS (computer) simulations of chemical plants and ran flow scenarios. I particularly enjoyed this modeling as if I were playing a computer game. I had a good grasp of constraints and degrees of freedom and had a knack for troubleshooting.

I drew process and instrumentation diagrams (P&IDs), taking great pride in the details. In one particular job, I was in charge of all P&ID updates and running them through CAD (computer-aided drafting). The plant was several hundreds of pages of detailed A3 drawings. I absolutely loved this responsibility. I took joy in marking up changes on the master copies and checking off changes as they came back from CAD. I guess it was my meticulous nature. Everything had to be perfect, and this task was perfect for me. Within a short time, I knew every detail of that plant backward[27].

The other calculations I worked on weren't as exciting for me. I think I would've been happy enough to do them had I been able to take them home and work in peace and quiet, but in the overstimulation of the cubicles, they required mental energy that I didn't have, and I got frequent headaches from trying to concentrate.

I struggled to focus on the work and yet remain aware enough of the people and conversations around me to maintain an illusion of normality. When someone suddenly laughed loudly or spoke to me, it would snap me out of what I was focusing on, and I would have urges to yell at them. (I made sure that it didn't show.) The computer gave me serious eye strain.

As someone who enjoys planning, I had a little more motivation when I was in control of a larger job from start to finish and could organize my time to suit me. But for the most part, the work was one random calculation after another. I was exhausted and struggled to keep going and going. I needed to escape.

---

[27] This is a saying that means to know something very well.

Within a month of starting, I began to dread going to work. On the train heading in, I would have dreams about the train crashing and sending me to hospital or the city being bombed (preferably overnight while empty of people!). I became depressed and numb Monday to Friday and spent most of Sunday crying, feeling ill because I had to go to work again the next day. I was in no way "okay."

When I mentioned it to people, I frequently got nonchalant replies such as, "Yeah, nobody likes working, but we all have to do it." So after a while, I learnt to stop complaining. At the time, I had no idea that I had Asperger's. And while I always had the sense that it must be worse for me than for other people, I couldn't justify that feeling.

Some months into the job, I started talking to my boss about not being happy in the role. I was trying to approach the issue with solutions, so I focused mainly on what it was about the work I wanted to change. I hadn't yet figured out that the environment was moreso the cause of those feelings. The feelings confused me, and I couldn't rationalize them. My boss seemed to want to be helpful, but he couldn't come up with much. I suspect he didn't understand the problem. Heavens, how could he? I didn't even understand the problem, so this went on for a long time.

During this job, I remember one particular incident that had a big impact on me. I think I was being myself a bit too freely one day and happened to make a childish, silly, and perhaps (unintentionally) inconsiderate remark among colleagues. My boss had a word to me privately. He told me—in a kind way—that I needed to think before I spoke. While he knew that I was capable and intelligent, others who didn't know me might form opinions that perhaps I was silly or odd, which would reduce their confidence in my work. I needed to present a professional image.

I took the criticism seriously. It was yet another reinforcement that being myself wasn't acceptable and that changing my behavior was going to be necessary for my success in life. How I wish I could go back now to undo these lessons and choose happiness instead.

At one point during this time, I suggested to my boss that I might like a transfer to a role in document control (managing P&IDs and other engineering drawings). He laughed and told me I was far too qualified for such a position. I still genuinely think it could've been a good place for me!

About a year and a half in, my boss suggested that maybe a transfer to safety and risk might suit me better. I was skeptical but felt pressured to take the role. I noticed about this time that I wasn't included in one of the usual training courses that I'd expected to go on. I think my discontentedness was making my boss nervous.

I asked if I could perhaps work part time. I had a feeling that I might be able to handle work better with some more time in between to rest and relax and do my own things. I was told no. If I was given that, then others might want it too. The company couldn't afford that. After all, what made me any different from anyone else? I think back now, if only I had known that I had Asperger's at the time, perhaps they could've made an exception.

As expected, the role in safety and risk didn't sit well with me at all, as it wasn't black and white like the usual engineering but grey and open ended with many possible answers to each problem. The group was also a bit short on work, and, for periods, my new boss, Trevor, asked me to just wait and "act busy" sometimes for days at a time. I had no idea how to make myself look busy when I wasn't. It was torturous trying to, and I'm not really good at acting and faking my way through things.

I remember one particular day walking into Trevor's office to ask what I could do for the fifty millionth time. It was hard on me to just sit there and keep my numbing mind contented while looking busy. I guess it must've been hard on him too to be repeatedly pressured to come up with work, because as I got near the door, I caught a glimpse of him in my peripheral vision. He'd ducked down behind the cubicle walls and was running away.

If I wasn't feeling down, I would've said it was quite a laughable thing to see a senior manager looking fancy in his formal suit scooting along the ground. After that, I just resigned myself to sitting at my desk and trying not to ask him what to do quite so much.

Eventually, when I could no longer stand it, I quit. I'd been trying to make it two years in the role, thinking that was approximately how much experience I would need to be generally "employable" should I ever want to come back. But at nineteen months, I decided that was close enough. Trevor accepted my resignation, as I think he didn't know what else to do with me. I was told that the company was happy with my quality of work and I was most welcome to come back if I ever wanted to. Of course, I never did. And so that ends the first chapter of my time as a full-time employee.

Chapter Seventeen

"Safe" versus "Unsafe" People

And now on to one of my more unusual trains of thought . . .

I was thinking the other day that as far back as I can remember, I've had this funny tendency to assess and categorize the people that I meet as either "safe" or "unsafe," which I'm aware is perhaps not a fair thing to do. But it's so intuitive, I'm not sure I could easily stop!

That might have you thinking, "Hang on. What do you mean by 'unsafe'? That doesn't sound like a nice thing to assume about somebody." But of course, when I say someone feels unsafe, I don't mean I think the person is bad in any way or a physical danger. I'm not talking about the good guys versus the bad guys or cops-and-robbers stereotypes.

It's more just a subtle sense I get of, "Can I trust this person to be accepting and positive toward me? Do I need to stress about my words and censor myself for fear of being taken the wrong way, or can I just relax and assume this person will try to 'get' me and not judge the things I do and say without first understanding?" It's a measure of kindness of spirit and how quickly I find myself comfortable around them.

And reading online recently, I noticed something rather surprising. It seems that a lot of Aspies out there are making comments about doing the same thing! I guess many of us can just feel in our gut who will be kind and who won't.

It made me wonder, is it like an extra sense we develop due to our vulnerability to political and social aggression? An ability to sniff out those who are well meaning from those who are inclined to judge, compete, and belittle? Or is it merely something that everyone detects but typical people don't seem to resist as much? Perhaps non-Autistics are more likely to put up with it because they value other qualities in individuals more highly, such as having someone to side with or popularity by association.

Either way, social politics have never moved me, so I'm more likely to choose the friends who give me that comfortable, at-ease, trusting vibe, and I'll go out of my way to surround myself with only people like that.

This prickly attitude of mine, however, does create some problems when it comes to complete strangers. Strangers. Yes, evil, scary strangers whom I haven't even really acknowledged yet or had time to "sniff out." You know the type. They lurk in corridors waiting to chat to you, the unsuspecting victim. You find them at malls, shops, restaurants, driving in cars, and even out on the streets. They're everywhere. Argh! Run for your Aspie life!

But no. In all honesty, I know I don't give strangers a fair chance. I'm aware that I should make more attempts to acknowledge them and get to know them better, but I just find it so hard to be around those I'm not familiar with.

Their reactions aren't easy for me to read and predict the way a friend's would be. Similarly, they don't know me well enough to interpret me easily, and I have to tread with more caution and turn that NT[28] simulator of mine way up! It drains energy, you know! So if I'm in anything but an energetic mood, I may ignore them a little more than is sociable. Sorry, stranger people. I don't mean to be rude, but sometimes you're just too tiring for me!

In the shops, when I'm most worn down, I'm—rather comically—known by my friends to be the one who's most likely to complain about the passersby. "Honestly, who let all these people in? Don't they know they're in my way? The shops would be so much more pleasant if someone got rid of them all!" Of course, I say this tongue-in-cheek, knowing very well that they have just as much right to be there as I do.

Out at dinner, when people come up to me to chat and I'm just not in the mood, I smile politely, nod, chat back, and think, "Go away. I'm busy. Can't you talk to someone else?" But look, see, I'm learning from typical people to hold my tongue. Once upon a time, I'd have said that out loud!

However, more realistically, I know that in order to even make friends, you have to sometimes give new people a chance, and if I'm talking to someone I'm likely to see in the future, I do try and kick myself in the butt and make the effort. After all, it would be impossible to function in the world or have any friends if I never got my act

---

[28] NT = neurotypical

together that way. And sometimes—just sometimes—I'm even lucky enough to get to know someone I like, which is always a pleasant surprise and certainly not what I expect at the onset! Who knew? Some of those evil, scary, unwelcome strangers actually turn out to be great people!

I know it's a shock, but nice people are out there. There may even be lots of them!

CHAPTER EIGHTEEN

ASPERGER'S AND EMPATHY

Q: So I'm confused. Do people with Asperger's have empathy or not?

Well, isn't that the big question that comes up over and over again?

I was having a good chat with a few Aspie friends of mine just yesterday at lunch-time over the topic of Asperger's and empathy. A small group of us with a bit of an interest in Aspie psychology decided we want to get together on a regular basis to talk about life and Aspie-related issues. We have been calling ourselves "The League of Extraordinary Aspies" (or "The League" for short) and have even formed a private Facebook group to coordinate our meetups, or secret little gatherings as I like to call them. I've been having some fascinating conversations with the group on all sorts of topics, and I'm really looking forward to our future chats!

Anyhow, after a rather long discussion with my new League friends, I think we came to some interesting conclusions yesterday on what we think empathy means for us Aspies. The crux of which I think was basically this: While we Aspies may admit-tedly be a little lacking in natural empathy and ability to pick up others' emotions, we are by no means lacking in compassion. And compassion is, after all, the heart of what people really want when they describe one another as empathetic or not. (So my apolo-gies to the League members from that week for stealing the group ideas!)

Now, to avoid confusion, I'll go ahead now and bring up the dictionary defini-tions that were mentioned in our group chat. Yes, you heard right. We had gathered for a fun, informal social chit chat, and someone pulled out a dictionary! That's Aspies for you!

So take a deep breath and prepare yourself for some dictionary-style text.

1. Compassion

Compassion is defined as: *"sympathetic pity and concern for the sufferings or misfortunes of others."*

So the word "compassion" seems to be a measure of where your heart is when others go through things—how deeply you care about those around you and those you love. And when I look around at my friends in the League, it's pretty clear to me that all of us demonstrate compassion. We care about the people in our lives and want them to do well, and it concerns us when our loved ones are having hard times.

I personally would consider myself to be strongly compassionate toward those whom I am close to, and having had my own negative experiences in life, I feel for others going through the same. I want to make life better for people. I believe it's immoral to intentionally hurt others in any way, even in subtle ways such as belittling, slighting, and excluding, and I think several other League members were similarly sensitive.

2. Empathy

Empathy, on the other hand, is defined as: *"the ability to understand and share the feelings of others."*

And this, I admit, is where we fall down, with the problem word being *share*. I think most Aspies do have a decent ability to understand the feelings of others on a logical and analytical level. But actually feeling them ourselves doesn't come naturally. I know when typical people listen to a story about another person's experience, they can have an immediate gut feeling of the emotions the other person is conveying. It can even be overwhelming for them.

Whereas when someone tells me a story, it's more a case of me thinking about it and deducing what the other person might be feeling. I don't automatically feel what they feel. I have to puzzle it out. Unfortunately, sometimes I don't put the pieces together until later, after the person has well and truly moved on in the conversation. Then it's too late to act empathetic.

An Aspie friend and family counselor I know, Grayson, once introduced me to the concept of mirror neurons, which are special nerves in our brains that help us automatically feel what another person would be feeling. For example, if a male were to see another man get kicked in the crotch, he might feel the urge to flinch too.

I don't know. It seems like an odd, hocus-pocus concept to me. But anyway, he was explaining that the latest research has indicated that perhaps Aspies, or *some* Aspies, don't have the same mirror neurons as typical people. So we lack the ability to instinctively feel what those around us might be feeling.

And—just privately—I can't even decide if this is a bad thing or a good thing, because it does offer us some protection from suffering along with those around us! For me, I know it makes me an easy friend to vent to, because I can care without feeling so drained by going through the emotional experiences myself that others tell me about. So I can tolerate a lot more.

If someone offered to come install mirror neurons in me, I think I'd run away screaming. No, thanks. I'm already drowning in my own emotions. I definitely don't need the addition of everyone else's on top of that! And I'm used to things this way, as strange as it may seem to all you normal-brained people out there! I don't want it to change.

So I guess that does make a strange combination of me caring but not always connecting in the typical way that others are used to. And this difference, unfortunately, can be easily misunderstood. But let me say one more time, just to bring the point home, that just because we Aspies don't feel the emotions of others strongly and always act thoughtfully does *not* mean that we don't care or have emotions ourselves. Of course we do. And hearing people imply such things can be rather offensive, really. Show some empathy, people!

Of course, with that comment there, I was half-joking. Well, doing one of those jokes that's sort of a joke, but not really . . . Because, more seriously, it can be quite upsetting to hear someone listing my actions and making accusations that I do things differently because I don't care, which I'm not just saying hypothetically. I actually had one person in my life recently do exactly that. And I wonder how they think that makes me feel.

It's almost a form of bullying to have someone telling you all the superficial things you do wrong and implying malice when there are simply no bad intentions there. It's crazy-making stuff, and I'm sure many Aspies out there have gone through it.

Now, having said all that and argued against the idea of Aspies lacking empathy, of course, now I'm going to turn around one hundred eighty degrees and admit that there's one area where I've noticed I am less empathetic than others. (I know, I'm a traitor! I'm admitting it out loud.) And that seems to be in having empathy for strangers or people I don't know a lot about.

I've always had a hard time understanding why people get so emotional over people in stories they read or hear about through word of mouth. Logically, to me, these stories are statistics. People die every day, and I find them sad and a shame or unfair to the person involved. But they've never really moved me the way they do others.

I can recall a few instances where I've had a bit of an "Aspie moment" in this regard. One day, I was waiting for a return email from a friend in order to organize events and hadn't heard back. At length, I received an email saying something along the lines of, "I'm sorry I haven't written sooner. My grandmother became suddenly ill, and we had to rush her to hospital. I've spent most of the morning there. I'll get back to you in the evening when I get home."

I have a tendency to scan for relevant facts and read it as "Sorry I haven't written. [insert reason here] Get back to you in the evening." So I replied along the lines of, "No worries. We'll sort it out in the evening."

Later that day, when Robert (my then husband) got home, I recounted to him, "We're not going to hear from Nik until a bit later. Something about his grandmother being sick or dying. Oh, I can't remember." To which Robert replied, "Oh, no. Nik and his grandma were very close." And that's when the penny dropped.

I got straight back on my email and wrote to him, saying, "Sorry I replied in a hurry before. How is your grandmother doing? Is she going to be okay?" Fortunately, my friend Nik never seemed to notice the insensitivity.

The problem that occurred here was that I somehow failed to perceive that my friend might be upset over this. I don't know how. Of course a person would be upset when someone they're close to falls ill. And he spent the day at the hospital, so of course this was someone whom he cared about. I should've known. But somehow, I just missed that one. My Aspie mind was too focused at the time on what we were trying to organize.

Sometime later, when my same friend posted a farewell online to his dog that had died, I felt that one strongly. I've had a dog of my own die. My "baby" Labrador retriever, Skye, was a close companion to me for sixteen years, perhaps my best friend as a child. I think of all the time I spent with her—her little personality quirks, how she used to cry if I left her to go into a shop and act absurdly excited when I came back out again as if she hadn't seen me for a year. I know what that feels like. So I could somehow relate to the grief one feels at the loss of a dog, but I've never had a person die when I was old enough to be moved in the same way. (Thankfully!)

Sometimes, when I think about Aspie empathy, I remember the events of September 11, 2001 and how I guess my reaction was different from most others'. I recall early that morning, seeing the news telecast about two planes crashing into buildings, terrorists, footage of the primary crash, etc., I thought, "Oh no, that isn't good," and then went on with my plans for the day.

Later in the day, I suddenly became aware that this was a big deal to people. Everyone seemed to be talking about it. People were emotional—unusually emotional. And yet, this same subset of people watch news of horrific car accidents weekly and don't seem to react. I thought the status quo was to ignore bad news and not think about it. Why was this different?

With 9/11, were they personally feeling for every victim of the impact? Was it the sheer size of the impact? When so many die at once, is the emotional buildup too much to bear? Or was it the involvement of terrorists creating fear? Fear perhaps that this could happen to them? The terror that the victims must have felt? And yet I have to argue that some of those life-and-death car accidents would be pretty terrifying for those involved as well. I never got my answers to these questions. Sometimes, the way others behave confuses me to no end!

Now, speaking about death—just to raise a topic in the blunt, ill-chosen, Aspie way—I just remembered another awkward Aspie moment I had involving my in-laws one day. My mother-in-law had a close personal friend named Jeanie who had been a family friend for many years. Robert was also close with her, although I'd only met her a couple of times. Sadly, Jeanie battled cancer and deteriorating health for some years.

One day when I logged on to my email, I saw a rather down message from my mother-in-law telling us the bad news that Jeanie had passed away. I had other things occupying my mind, so it didn't really sink in for me, and I didn't know what to say in reply. I don't generally know how to reply to these things! So I thought, "Uh oh, I'll leave that one for Robert to deal with," and I moved on. Unfortunately, I didn't notice that the email had been addressed only to me.

Perhaps a week later, my mother-in-law called and asked if I'd passed on the bad news. I was stumped. I hadn't. I'd completely forgotten about it, which I think surprised her. In fact, I was lucky I didn't reply, "What bad news?" I suppose the typical thing to do after getting the initial email would've been to spend at least an evening with Robert lamenting how sad the whole thing was. She was certainly someone Robert was close to, and it should have at least resonated with him. But it hadn't occurred to me to bring it up.

I wonder how others judge me when I do more serious things like this. What they interpret it to mean. I don't have any ill intentions when I do it. This is just how empathy is for me. I need to establish it logically. I try to tune in and think about how others are reacting to things. I want to be supportive, but if I'm preoccupied with something else, then sometimes I do miss things, and I can't be running at 100 percent and fully tuned in all the time. I do my best, but I'm human, after all. (Which is really the most ironic part!)

CHAPTER NINETEEN

BLACK-AND-WHITE MORALS

Q: I've heard that people with Asperger's are often described as having a good sense of morality compared to typical people. Do you?

Umm . . . Well, I would have to say yes! Morality is an interesting topic and one that I definitely have opinions on. I think, going back, I've always had a strong, black-and-white sense of right and wrong, even at those stages in my life when I was sure that I knew everything but didn't have a clue! (You know those good old teen years.)

When I was young, I recall being very concerned about people following the rules as I perceived them, and sometimes I was perhaps bossy and meticulous about it. People straying was not acceptable, and the rules had to be what I thought they were! But I think that is a little bit the Aspie way. Fancy that, an Aspie child being over the top about rule following and needing things to be their way!

As I've grown up and matured, however, I've learned that real life comes in shades of grey. There are many situations far too complex to fit into simple black and white boxes, and each case needs to be evaluated on its own merits. Strict adherence to "the rules," I think, becomes less important than human welfare when facing real-life people who need empathy and understanding.

For example, how would you react to a friend who, say, chose to terminate a midterm pregnancy when you didn't really comprehend why or know the struggles she went through to make that decision? What if she came to you for help? (I know—a controversial issue for some!) To me, that one is easy.

Nowadays, I still have a strong moral conscience, but I've moved more toward be-lieving true morals are a measure of how well and respectfully you treat those around you rather than just being about following rules. I'm all about maximizing the happi-ness and well-being of myself and others and minimizing harm to anything, really—people, animals, the environment, etc.

It's a simple concept, but sometimes it takes a lot more pondering to figure out what's right and wrong under this broader framework, and not everyone can be that much of a thinker. So I do understand why some would be more comfortable having rules to fall back on. It also requires you to truly value others and think about their perspectives and not just your own. Wow, how far I've come as an Aspie there!

I do my best, and I feel a sense of peace with my views on life and humanism (the idea of people focusing on helping each other out). And personally, I don't think I could live under any other philosophy and still feel honest and true to myself as a person. But each to their own, as we all view the world in *very* different ways and have our own philosophies on life and what we think is right and wrong.

On a side note, a friend of mine, Josh, once posed a question to me that I thought was interesting (paraphrased):

If there were no other life forms on Earth, is there anything you could do that would be wrong?

I think the answer is no, but it certainly gets you thinking and makes a good topic for discussion . . .

Chapter Twenty

My Second Full-Time Job, Valcorp Technical Centre

And now to go back into my story about life as a working Aspie:

After having left my job at Worley, I was a little reluctant to enter the workforce in a conventional way again. I came up with dream ideas of ways I could work for myself. I pictured sewing and selling baby clothes on Ebay. I'd only ever sewn two garments before and had no real idea about it at all, but it was one of those ideas that appealed to me. Any business management idea appeals to me, really. I pictured the whole enterprise, planning it in my head, right down to how I would manage inventory and coordinate shipping to be reliable.

Robert pointed out to me that with market competition, I would be unlikely to make any money this way. I wasn't exactly planning on running a sweatshop. I did the maths roughly and had to agree with him. That idea died.

I started to look into franchises and small business opportunities, but this idea faded even more quickly than the first when I reasoned that we would make just as much money investing the capital than the likely return on a business, and with far less effort and risk.

In the meantime, I scanned the papers and the internet for other employment opportunities. Robert insisted that the most sensible thing for me to do at this point was to work for an employer like everyone else. I had no specific expertise that would allow me to break out on my own nor any real product to sell. Perhaps another working role would suit me better than the first had if I found the right one.

And so, I reluctantly agreed, only because at the time, working the conventional way seemed to be the only socially acceptable thing to do, given my lack of other options. How could I justify myself to the world if I wasn't a career person?

Now that I look back, I think it's a great shame that I felt so forced to do something that makes me so unhappy solely because of social pressures. What has the world come to that job status and wealth feel like they're more important to a person than who we are as people and the things that we love and that inspire us? The world is backward. Society's rules are rigid. The business-world structure works for the majority, but for those of us for whom it doesn't, the alternatives are scarce.

When I think about me and who I am, there are so many other ways I could contribute to society if only it were flexible enough to allow me to slowly find a way to do it that works for me. I'm not being "lazy" in not wanting to have a nine-to-five job. It just doesn't work for me. It seems okay for other people, but not for me. Am I the only person in the world that has ever felt this way?

So, back to the job hunt. I decided this time that I wanted to apply for a job in plastics, as I'd always found the plastics industry a little more interesting. It brought back images of me as a child playing with plastic resin that my father had brought home from work, digging little tunnels and moving around the beads that my parents had used to fill potholes in the driveway.

At this point, I still failed to understand where exactly my difficulties in the workforce were stemming from, so I reasoned that maybe if the field of work interested me enough, I could find that extra bit of motivation to get me through the days. Logic, logic, logic. I can see why finding a workplace fit is so much simpler for people who just go by feelings! I was way off track.

I also decided that there was no way I was going to work in an office cubicle environment again. At least that one was based on gut. I wanted a site job where I could walk around and see and touch things—real things, not just paper and computer screens all day. So in interviews, I cited my reason for leaving Worley as wanting a more "hands-on" job. This was not untrue in itself.

It didn't take me long to find a job in a plastics research and development site. The first role that came up cited spending a lot of time working at the company sites, so it seemed a good fit, given my logical job criteria, and before I knew it—less than a month after I had quit Worley—I'd started work at my new job. It all happened so fast, I never had time to stop and rest or think about what I wanted. I had one idea, and then straight away, I was snapped up into the workforce again.

So I packed myself up and moved house to a little apartment up north where the new role was located. Robert, whom I was due to marry in a matter of months, planned to come live with me up at the site once his work role changed, presumably a year before we were married. In reality, that role change took much longer than expected—his work did things like that!—and it wasn't until several months after our marriage that we got to actually live together for the first time. We had our wedding ceremony, and then after only a few short days together, we drove off back to our separate houses three hours' drive apart. Talk about a strange start to a marriage!

My boss at my new job, Kurt, was actually a great guy. He was a people person and liked to grow and encourage each individual working under him. Our team was small. In the plastics section, it was just myself and Tony—a much more experienced colleague—and then there was also Aaron working in cans and beverage.

Kurt noticed quickly that I seemed to be reluctant in some of the tasks he set me. He was in tune to those types of behaviors and assumed I was lacking in confidence, so he set about trying to give me as much exposure to "people" tasks as possible—throwing me in the deep end for my own good, so to speak. He nudged me into a few jobs such as ringing around to find out information, talking to suppliers, organizing logistics for trials, and generally going out and talking to strangers to establish networks and discuss opportunities. He was so well intentioned and determined to help break me out of my shell, but little did he know he was torturing me!

Having both social anxiety and Asperger's Syndrome, the overstimulation and discomfort of doing these tasks was making me feel sicker than I ever had. I mostly found ways to avoid them, but with Kurt "encouraging" me, more and more, I was forced to suck it down and do them.

He really was only trying to compel me to grow and show me how things were done. He insisted on trying to "broaden" me and give me exposure to constant new sites and types of work, as he felt it would help my bigger-picture development. But I insisted I just wanted to settle down and become an expert in one thing. I liked to do the same work over and over and wanted a simple life. Kurt didn't really buy it and felt sure he could eventually get through to me and help me achieve better. It was sort of a battle of willpower between two people both coming from a good place.

On top of that, I was still suffering from those same feelings I'd experienced in my last job. They seemed to be "of unknown origin."

I had learnt from my Worley experience not to complain too much about disliking my work. It didn't achieve anything positive. So I didn't try to discuss my feelings as much with Kurt.

The constant stress was giving me stomach upsets, and my weight plummeted down to 52kg (110 lb) at the lowest (I am 5'7"). When my cycles stopped, I went to see a doctor, who ordered a series of tests. It all came back fine except that perhaps my stress levels were high. The doctor told me that I was underweight and gave me a lecture on "work-life balance." My god, if only it were that simple!

At the same time, I started spending a lot of time with my colleague Tony. He was more like me than anyone else I'd ever met, and we hung back after work and had long, deep conversations. I have no doubt that Tony sits somewhere on the Asperger's spectrum himself, and in an email conversation many years later, he agreed, though his ability to cope with the world was strong where mine was not.

Tony was respected by those around him and known for his self-assured, honest, no-nonsense attitude. His quirkiness, humor, and "mafia-like" style of saying shocking but true things were highly regarded by everyone who met him. He was comfortable within himself and had no problem with doing things his way, regardless of what others thought. Other people moved out of his way and let him do his thing.

Less than a year into my new job, Tony was recruited by one of the plastics plants directly, and shortly after, he let me know that there was a technical role under him that I might like to transfer to. I jumped at the opportunity to change jobs, if only to get out of the push-pull of having to do such stressful little social tasks!

I remember my last feedback session with Kurt. He made the comment that it was the first time we had had feedback without me crying, and I responded quickly that it was because I knew I was leaving. Unfortunately, I think I might've insulted him with that, as after all, he'd tried hard to do a lot for me.

What was really going on, of course, was that in every feedback session, Kurt would talk to "motivate" me into doing tasks, and at some point, I would realize that I was inevitably going to have to do them. There was no way of avoiding it. Each time, this created that sinking feeling, causing me to end up stressed and tearful. I liken it to the feeling a gunman might feel if they suddenly realized they had to shoot someone they know.

Of course, no one was forcing me, but in my mind, I didn't understand that I had choices. All my life, I'd done what I was told. It was my permission to be.[29] That last session, I knew I was leaving and would be able to avoid the worst of the tasks that Kurt had set for me. I was relieved.

Kurt's response to me leaving was to tell me that he didn't think I was "ready" (presumably to cope with real-life site politics and people). He said it in a way that sort of offended me, knowing that I was at least technically competent. Not that he was impolite or snarky about it, I just didn't know what he was implying by that. In hindsight, I think he was actually right. I wasn't ready for the social politics of the new site. But Kurt's methods of "readying" me were never going to succeed, so that was a dead end too, and I couldn't have run away fast enough.

---

[29] My "permission to be" is a term I've come across in counselling. (Psychology lingo.) For someone with low self-esteem, it can be what they believe they have to be or do just to be acceptable and earn the right to exist. For me, for many years, I felt like being perfect, doing what I was told, and doing everything right was my permission to be.

In the end, Kurt never threw a farewell for me like he did Tony. I guess he felt awkward or disgruntled about the way I'd handled things. And in hindsight, I don't really blame him!

Chapter Twenty-One

Kindness and Understanding on the Spectrum

So, going back to one of those random trains of thought of mine . . .

Over the last few months, I've been spending a lot more time with other Aspies than I ever have in my life. Heavens, until about a year ago, I didn't even know such people existed! And just the other day, it hit me that as a group, there's something really genuine and beautiful about our Aspie behavior.

It's something I sense immediately when I walk into an Aspie gathering that's hard to describe, but it jumps out in an unmistakable way. Perhaps it's in the way we're so naturally open and sincere as opposed to gravitating toward manipulative, bitchy, or competitive behaviors. Perhaps it's in the way we truly mean what we say and are happy to see our friends and colleagues do well. We don't act or fake our behavior due to hidden agendas. We're not inclined toward pretense. We have no drive to seek power over others or mistreat others. It's really a case of what you see is what you get, and you can trust in that.

I remember first having this realization during a League meeting one evening when listening to a guy in the group, Josh, describe how, while growing up, he typically "turned enemies into friends" by reacting with humor and understanding to their misguided behaviors. It showed a high level of introspection and drive to accept even the most troublesome people from a young age—a level of maturity above what one would normally expect.

I can't remember all the replies to the conversation now, but it gave me the sense that our group, on the whole, had similar tendencies, the common theme being that we're strongly compassionate people who naturally want to understand, mediate, and make peace when friction arises.

I suppose, having grown up as Aspies, we've all had to work hard at relationships and see working to understand others, even in periods of bad behaviors, as part of what friendship is. And, as a consequence, we're more forgiving than most. I'm not sure if this sort of tolerance is common to all Aspies, but it's certainly a theme I've seen in the most mature of us, and it made me wonder if it was reflected in the Aspie population at large.

I know, for me, that when a person says unkind things, I don't focus on the words they're saying. I focus on why they are saying it and what emotions and issues in themselves are driving it. It's amazing when I do this how frequently I discover that the real source of their negativity isn't even about me. Understanding how people tick makes it so much easier to be compassionate at these times.

I have a good example of this involving a relative, Amanda, at the time when we were both pregnant with our first babies. (And Amanda, please don't kill me for writing about this! It was just too interesting an example to pass up.)

Shortly after having an ultrasound that revealed the sex of my son, I sent out a generic text to family and friends announcing how happy my husband and I were to be expecting a boy. Amanda wrote back a positive response expressing her happiness for us, to which I replied, "Yes, we are over the moon." About a minute later, I received a further text from her saying, "Apparently she is over the moon. I wish she would go over the other side of the moon! Literally."

For a second, the text confused me, but I realized quite quickly that it had been sent to the wrong person and that she was, in fact, having a dig at me. I stopped to think about it for a few minutes, then replied, "That was a strange text to receive."

Several minutes on, Amanda called me on the phone, upset. She said she was so sorry and that the text was intended for her husband. She didn't seem to want to spell it out in case I'd missed the meaning. I asked her, "What about me having a boy upset you so much?" to which she burst into tears.

She explained that she was jealous of me being pregnant with a boy and how much it meant to her to be able to give her husband a son to carry on the family name. He's the last in his line. She only ever wanted to have two kids, and she had a fear about having two girls. She didn't know the gender of her own baby yet, and apparently, it had been stressing her a lot.

Upon listening to her talk, it became clear to me that the aggression she had shown was not really about me at all but an expression of her own insecurities. Sometimes, people do lash out at the wrong person when something makes them emotional. Understanding this, any anger I had at her comment disappeared. I felt sorry for her and sorry that this issue was causing her so much stress.

I said to her, "I don't like that you wrote that, but I think we can let it go and move forward." Of course, when I say we can move forward, I actually mean it in the Aspie way, that I really have let it go. It doesn't mean I plan to hold on to the emotion and make snipes back from time to time or bring it up in arguments like some people can. On the contrary, it means I'm now able to move forward with positive feelings.

So we did, and Amanda and I became much closer from the interaction. Perhaps it improved her opinion of me because it showed her my capacity to be understanding and forgiving, someone with that kind and beautiful Aspie nature I've described.

I think a lot of Aspies have these beautiful natures, but it almost takes a combative incident for others to see it in us and be able to truly value how sweet a friend we can be. Unfortunately, being open-minded and accepting of others are not traits that society judges us on when forming early impressions. Too often, we're dismissed for superficial characteristics up front, without people ever really getting to know us and see what extraordinary people we are inside.

Then again, I've also seen quite a few Aspies who are jaded and angry about their life experiences and too caught up in that to have really learnt to view others in a mature way. And I've definitely seen Autistic meltdowns and reactive behavior under stress. So maybe I'm way off base on this topic . . . or maybe not. It's just my miscellaneous thought for the day, so I'll leave it to you to decide what to make of it.

CHAPTER TWENTY-TWO

BEING "GIFTED"

Q: So what do you think are the positive elements to being an Aspie? I've heard some people talk about Aspies being talented. Is there any truth to that?

Oh, yes! When I think about my Asperger's nowadays, I realize just how lucky I am to have this "syndrome," because the strengths that come with it really are something I value.

Being socially awkward, "quirky," different, "weird," "inappropriate," sometimes isolated, and not fitting into the nine-to-five role, this is the price I pay for the talents I've landed. In the wrong environment, it can be a real struggle, but in the right nurturing one, it's so worth the prize.

I recently heard a quote from Tony Attwood pointing out that "most of the major advances in science and art have been made by people with Asperger's Syndrome,"[30] which is outstanding, really, considering how rare Asperger's is in the population! Understanding Asperger's the way I do, it doesn't surprise me. We have minds that are designed for great contribution. We're the deep thinkers and inventors of the world!

---

[30] Tony Attwood, Quoted in: Wine, Angela, "About Asperger's Syndrome," 2006, http://www.aspergerkid.com/about_AS.html

Tony Attwood went on to say, "Asperger's has probably been an important and valuable characteristic of our species throughout evolution."[31] And I have to agree. I wonder if, without Aspies, the human race could have advanced as rapidly as it has. I cherish my hyperfocus and deep thinking. I would hate to have been born any other way.

As individuals, of course, we do vary greatly. Every one of us has different interests, strengths, and modes of thinking which can lead to very different focuses. Some of us have extremely strong interests in more common areas such as math, science, engineering, literature, music, drawing, painting, photography, acting, programming, etc. However, this focus could go anywhere: studying oscillating fans, recreating corporate logos, collecting topological maps, and so on.

I've heard of some Aspies who excel in many areas and some who don't really excel in anything in particular, bar perhaps playing games or having extensive knowledge of TV shows. But you know, that's the way life works out. Things are always a little random.

I myself think that having hyperfocus in our pocket—for the majority of us who do—can be a huge advantage to almost any task. When we tackle problems of interest, we can do it with intense concentration, repetition, and persistence.

Unlike typical people, we're not afraid to be left alone with our item of interest for long periods of time to get things done. We will persevere for as long as a task takes, even sometimes forgoing meals or social engagements—whatever it takes to achieve an outcome to our level of satisfaction! Believe me, I know what it's like to get too caught up to eat. I'm usually only reminded when I start to feel a bit sick and my tummy reminds me. Oh, that's right. I haven't eaten in eight hours. I forgot!

But, so as not to give all the credit to hyperfocus, we also do have a few other cool things going for us: We're naturally detail oriented and can be great at seeing specifics that others may miss. We reason logically and methodically and can be "outside-the-box" problem solvers. And we really enjoy forming a deep base of knowledge in our specialty areas, which makes us likely to become experts in our field.

Heck, once we get going on something, we can be surprisingly visionary about what we want to achieve, well above and beyond what's usual. I know that once I have a concept in mind, I become ridiculously eager to stop everything else I'm doing and plan it out in detail then and there from the big picture right down to weird, unimportant details that my mind comes up with, such as how I am going to lay out my storage room. Planning is fun, and I wish I had such visions more often just for the simple joy of being able to map the ideas out!

---

[31] Tony Attwood, 2006, p2 Quoted in: Fattig, Michelle "Famous People with Aspergers Syndrome," Disabled World, 12/28/2007 http://www.disabled-world.com/artman/publish/article_2086.shtml

On top of all that, I've also heard of many Aspies having unique and creative talents in the arts, which, while not my area, is apparently a popular Aspie field. I guess it's unsurprising when you consider how different our minds and creative processes are from the norm! I can only imagine what random stuff a group of Aspies would come up with. The mind boggles. And maybe it's just the perfectionist in me talking, but I can see how being fussy about the details could also be a big advantage when shaping an artistic product.

For example, an Aspie artist who is fussy about specifics may work on his/her piece over and over until the work is "just right" according to his or her vision, altering details that others may not even notice. They may work on it long after others would have declared the job finished. I think Hans Asperger (the man after whom Asperger's Syndrome was named), originally described this phenomenon when he said, "For success in science or art, a dash of Autism is essential."[32] And there have certainly been many examples of Aspies in the history of the arts to back this up!

For example, here is a list of historical or famous people (across all fields) who are either known to or are now speculated to have had Asperger's based on their known personality traits:

- Albert Einstein
- Isaac Newton
- Bill Gates
- Abraham Lincoln
- Benjamin Franklin
- George Washington
- Charles Darwin
- George Mendel
- Carl Sagan
- Wolfgang Mozart
- Thomas Jefferson
- Marie Curie
- Henry Ford

- Marilyn Monroe
- Jane Austin
- Ludwig Van Beethoven
- Michelangelo
- Richard Strauss
- Thomas Edison
- Vincent Van Gough
- Virginia Wolf
- Alfred Hitchcock
- Bob Dylan
- Charles Dickinson
- Robin Williams

- Hans Christian Anderson
- James Maury "Jim" Henson
- George Orwell
- Dan Aykroyd
- Woody Allen
- Mark Twain

---

[32] Hans Asperger, Quoted in: Your Little Professor, "The Benefits of Asperger's Syndrome," (no date or author provided), http://www.yourlittleprofessor.com/benefits.html

You have to agree, that's quite an extensive list! But please don't quiz me on the details of these. I will admit I just got them from Google! Following celebrities has never been an interest of mine; however, feel free to look them up if you yourself are more fascinated with them than I am! After all, most people are.

And now, last but not least, while I'm on a roll here, I wanted to mention one more awesome thing about Aspies that most people don't think about very much. That is the many positive characteristics of our personality (social awkwardness aside). Though you may think of these as being nothing much, if you search the depths of the internet, there are actually a lot of great things that people have to say about us.

We've been described as honest, loyal, compassionate, non-judgmental, open minded, trusting, reliable, dependable, and caring to the significant people in our lives (although we don't always express it in conventional ways). We're rarely manipulative, bitchy, backstabbing, or fickle. We value others based on their behavior, not superficial attributes, and give all people a fair chance. Aspies can really make loyal, dependable friends to those who take the time to recognize those traits and treat us well.

So I can't speak for everyone, but personally, I'm so glad I was born an Aspie with all the logic, rationality, and other gifts that come with it, because it's such an important and special part of me. I like being able to question and analyze the world around me. I like being part of a group that philosophizes and even questions cultural rules, religions, politics, etc. We are the ones who challenge the society that we live in and question whether things are right.

Without this introspection and critical thinking, I wouldn't be me, and I wouldn't have been able to reach the levels of peace, understanding, and insight that I've achieved. And that's something I wouldn't trade for all the money in the world. Long live Aspie gifts!

Chapter Twenty-Three

My Third Full-Time Job, Valcorp Ringwood

And now to delve back into the story of my working life.

After finally getting away from the Technical Centre, my role at Valcorp Ringwood started on a positive note. I'd often gone down to the plastics plant when working at the Technical Centre, and I loved the excitement of how up-and-coming this little site was. New customers were being won. New machinery was being put in, and sales were set to boom. There was something about the little plastic-sheet-and-cup site that felt like home to me. Perhaps it was the nostalgia of running those little plastic pellets through my hands in my childhood—a very satisfying sensory experience.

Walking out around the plastics plant at Ringwood, I enjoyed seeing the familiar resin and product. I also got to wear ear muffs, which felt wonderful to someone like me. They eased my noise sensitivity and left me with just the rhythmic noises of the thermoformers playing in my head like a song. I wasn't stuck in an office cubicle anymore. That, to me, was bliss, and I was so relieved have been officially offered the job.

Going through the recruitment process to get this role had turned out to be tedious. It was several months after Tony had transferred to Ringwood that I had first heard the new technical position was available. One of the original staff, Justin, had either left or gotten fired—the details of which nobody seemed to want to tell me exactly—leaving open a vacancy for someone to do the process calculations and write operating settings for the extruder and thermoformer machinery.

In the past, they'd used experienced operators for that role. But this time around, Edward (the plant manager) and Tony had a different idea in mind. They wanted someone familiar with plastics but more intellectual who was able to learn and do more complex studies and trials to improve the products. Someone with a degree. And so Tony took me aside one day, before the role was announced, and gave me a heads up that, in his mind, I would be perfect for the job. He encouraged me to apply.

The recruitment process itself was unfortunately lengthy, requiring resumes and several interviews with existing staff—staff whom I already knew, which was odd. But eventually, after all applicants had been considered, I was finally deemed the best candidate and offered the role. Woohoo! Freedom! I had moved to an on-site job. It all had to be easier now, surely!

The new plant site, which I now had the joy of calling my own, felt warm and homey to me, with a little factory, warehouse, and office building that spread over about two acres. I mostly worked in the office, writing specifications for how new products would be run or planning trials for new materials, but I also spent time out on the factory floor learning the equipment and helping troubleshoot problems. My role was titled "Process Improvement Leader" and was a technical position working directly under Tony. In fact, Tony and I made up the whole technical team.

Out in the factory, we had one multilayer extrusion machine. Little resin pellets would drop into a series of six screw pumps, which melted the plastic and injected it into a block that layered and flattened the molten plastic into a sheet. The extruded sheet was then wound over a series of cooling rollers and past edge trimmers before being wound onto a roll.

We also had several thermoforming machines which took the rolls of sheet, heated it in massive heater banks, and then punched the plastic into cup molds to form ten or more cups at a time. One machine had conveyer belts with moving arms to stack the cups and run them past a quality-check camera. The cups were then automatically packed in a packing and bagging machine.

At any time, there were always several operators working on each line, testing the sheet and cup quality and adjusting minor equipment settings or wrapping and boxing cups and rolls of sheet. I quickly made friends with most of the regular operators and found a real fondness for wandering around the factory, discussing with people how the lines were running—plus engaging in the occasional blue-collar banter and mischief that we all enjoyed.

One day, a couple of the guys asked me to hold a hose for them, and I was naively standing still holding it when it suddenly poured buckets of water out of the cooling rollers all over my shirt and top. Hey, not funny, guys—although I have to admit underneath it really was. They got me good there. And so I spent my days wandering in and out whenever I felt that need for a break and some fun social time.

Back in the management quarters, I was set up promptly with a good-sized desk and computer in the main production office. And I have to say, our little office of five had some interesting characters.

Edward, the plant manager whom I mentioned before, liked to sit at the head of the room, looking like the lord of the office. He was a tall man who was surprisingly young and in good shape—certainly not the heavy, hairy old man you'd expect from a plant manager stereotype.

Often, for lunch, he would splurge by taking the entire team out to a café and talk to us over glorious-looking food about his philosophies for plant success. I think he fancied himself quite the people motivator and manipulator and would come out with lines such as, "Nobody is irreplaceable" and staff should give "110 percent." Although his philosophies were often a little too cutthroat and un-empathetic for my taste.

Sitting opposite to me in the main office, facing away, was Hugo, the production manager—a stern-looking man, who many others referred to as attractive, although I have to say he rather intimidated me a little, and I couldn't see him that way. It is hard to put my finger on exactly why I had trouble with him, but for some reason, I feared his disapproval, and every so often, when Hugo was around, I would embarrass myself by saying silly, nervous things or becoming extra clumsy. Reversing out of the car park one day into his shiny new blue utility vehicle was definitely a bad move! Almost crashing a 0.8 tonne roll of plastic into a thermoformer one day was another. Darn anxiety.

Though in Hugo's defense, he did take the car incident well, considering how much he loves his car, and accepted payment for the damage without fuss. Boy, was I glad his desk wasn't positioned to face mine!

Tony had been allocated the desk beside mine, and then . . . I suddenly realized I need to brashly interrupt my sentence with an introduction of Rosie and talk at length about Rosie *only*, as there would be no more fitting way to present her! An awkward, in-your-face prelude to her very special self. Oh my gosh, Rosie!

The final person in our office, Rosie, was a newly appointed quality manager at the plant who had quickly got herself involved with staffing rosters and any other major or staff decisions as well. She was a petite lady of slim build, which she really knew how to work to make herself noticed.

Rosie was extremely assertive, and what I really mean by that is "aggressive"— but shhh. Let's say assertive to be polite, as she *was* that too. She was able to be extremely loud when required and had a knack for keeping all the attention in the room on herself. Yet, paradoxically, most of the time, she was playful, smiley, and had a sweet, girlish, almost "innocent-if-you-didn't-know-her" demeanor. Sometimes, she felt sickly sweet to me, but most people like that.

When I was first interviewed for the position, Rosie had been positive toward the idea and had voted for me. She knew me a little from the times I'd come down to the site to help her with trials and performing quality checks on the cups, though I'd been more timid then, as she was still a stranger to me. She welcomed me with sweet smiles and words of warmth and made me feel at home on the team.

Settling into the management office at Ringwood—the office in which Rosie resided—I couldn't help but be amused (and sometimes gobsmacked) by her constant banter and sexual innuendo. A life-sized wooden penis ash tray stood up tall and proud on her desk. We referred to it as Woody, and oh, the fun the office had joking about that. Rosie's love life was supposedly lacking, and people made cheeky comments about how she needn't worry about getting pregnant because Woody was infertile.

Over the course of a day, Rosie talked about penises and men "cumming in their pants" and anything else crude with little hesitation in between sweet, ladylike conduct. It was usually done in a playful way and was hilarious for shock value. I was always fighting back tears of laughter when new people came by who didn't know her. Oh, the expressions on their faces! Such words from such a virtuous-looking little lady! Did they hear that right?

When Tony was recruited, apparently, she had joked about being part of his employment package. Little one-liners were thrown back and forth about him taking her off into a closet. Of course, it was always just suggestive talk and nothing more.

But anyway, moving on . . .

Working alongside this team, I quickly learnt my way around my new role. I realized early on that to keep the sheet running smoothly, I needed to spend a lot of time wandering around the extruders, checking for errors in the setup, and writing little notes to communicate to operators about any changes that were to be made. I hastily drew diagrams and made sense of the complex network of piping, dryers, and hoppers used for loading products and additives into the extruders and learnt to monitor what was going in where, where most of the errors occurred.

My role also involved going out to customer sites to help troubleshoot issues and talk about changes or improvements they wanted made to the sheet and/or cups. I have some fond memories of days out with Tony, studying the puree fruit lines at a company called Cirrup. Tony was fun to work with and made things feel leisurely. He invested a lot into training me and teaching me everything that he knew. It felt like the old Italian style—I scratch your back, you scratch mine.

In the middle of the trips, we would often find a place to go eat lunch while chatting about the amusing antics of the customers and people at our own site. I really looked forward to those lunches and the long car rides there and back through the rural Australian streets, with gum trees overhead and fields as far as the eye could see. I used to look up to see if I could spot koalas while we drove. So much about this role was great.

However, as I settled into the site and became comfortable, I started to notice that the politics in the office were complicated and hard to follow. Information at the site, for some reason, was treated like currency and not shared readily, even when it was important knowledge about machinery or plans for up-and-coming projects. It made it frustrating to communicate with people and get things done that needed doing.

I remember how often on our breaks, Tony and I would go outside to sit on the table outside, awash with a fog of cigarette smoke, and talk to those on "smoko" about what was going on at the site. Passive smoking was never something I enjoyed, but as one of the only two non-smokers on the site, it was either that or be left out of the loop. For such a pretty little lady, Rosie was surprisingly like a chimney and often sat there chit-chatting for lengthy periods at a time.

The other place that information was shared was the main management meetings that were held upstairs every morning, and at first, I had rather enjoyed sitting around the large oval table with the team and listening to the goings-on at the plant. However, only a few months in, Edward made a decision to reduce the number of people in the room and removed (only) me from attendance. He didn't require both me and Tony to be there at the same time.

After that, trying to understand the day-to-day goings-on of the plant really started to perplex me. I was never really one for going around and having words in people's ears and working to get information. I just wanted someone to tell me everything that was happening.

A little while in, perhaps after the first six months working there, I also noticed Rosie's attitude toward me slowly shifting from motherly to competitive, and she started being inconsistent in how she responded to me—sweet one minute, aggressive the next, and then back to sweet again as if nothing had happened.

One thing I do know is that she started to be constantly in Edward's ear like a little bird, whispering things to him about my supposed faults and errors to make herself look good. Edward always claimed to know what Rosie was like and to be able to ignore her attempts to influence him, but I'm sure that at least some things were slowly seeping in this way by the questions Edward would occasionally ask Tony and myself. Such as, why were we out for such a long lunch the other day?

At one point, it was brought to Edward's attention how supposedly incompetent I was at fixing a problem on the extrusion line, one I swore was a mechanical problem with the cooling roller that couldn't be fixed with process alone. A secret trial was conducted behind my back, where Rosie, Hugo, and Edward gathered one or two of their most experienced operators to fiddle with the sheet and try and fix the problem.

They tried for several hours, but fortunately for me, I guess, they couldn't make it any better either. Rosie also liked to go out and fiddle with the process settings on the line, showing off her supposed expertise to the operators. Whether it helped anything or not, I couldn't say, but she never did tell me what she'd changed, so it made it hard for me to do my job.

Later that year, out of the blue, I was suddenly told that I'd been removed from doing site visits, as Edward explained that Rosie's expertise would be more helpful out at site. At first, I was confused by the swap, but eventually, toward the end of my time at the plant, I had the real reason explained to me. Edward believed (or had been told) that if I couldn't even fix our own line, then what use would I be out at site? Apparently, I needed more training on our own equipment first. I wonder who convinced him of that.

Tony and Rosie went on a week's trip together to see a customer in New Zealand and had many days out at Cirrup and other local customer plants. I missed out on some fun times and felt trapped in a site where I'd already solved all that was in my capacity to solve. I wasn't a mechanical person and didn't really know what to do about the rollers. The situation was rotten.

I also found myself having a lot of trouble talking with Edward the way Rosie did. I always rather liked Edward's jovial, witty nature and would have wanted to be friends with him myself were it simple, but I never did figure out how to break the ice with him. I mean, I liked the guy, but we just couldn't communicate. I had trouble reading him and working out where I stood and when I was welcome to approach. And I think he was perplexed by me and my reactions to things. He couldn't predict me at all, which I'm sure must have been frustrating to him as someone who prized himself for knowing how to work others.

He seemed to respect me mostly when I did things that were bold and contrary to what you would expect. For example, one day—back in the time when I was based at the technical centre—Edward had stood me up for an appointment with him, and I pretty much told him off about poor time management. I commented that I don't have to come out and see him, and if he wanted my help, he needed to do better or at least have the courtesy to reschedule. Bold of me, I know! I think it took him aback, and instead of being offended, he acted like he loved the power I'd wielded on that day and rather admired the move.

Another day, around the same time period, Edward made a crass joke to my technical centre boss, Kurt, and me about whipping out his penis, and without hesitation, I enthusiastically remarked, "Come on, then. Show us." I remember how he turned a little red and stumbled out of the room for a minute before coming back in to talk business. I really called his bluff on that one, and he was just mesmerized every time someone outplayed him in any way. He always did confess to having a weakness for the ladies, so I think that sort of humor also appealed to him.

What a funny world to find myself in. How is an Aspie supposed to make sense of any of this, really?

Most of the time that I was at Ringwood, I found the antics of these people around me highly amusing. Often, when the plant management meetings were going on upstairs, I would hear Rosie's yelling coming down the staircase or heavy arguments being had over simple decisions. Things could get fiery. I remember one day how an operator from the floor, Finn, came into the office where I was sitting and rolled his eyes at me to indicate the ridiculousness of what was being said. But I just laughed that sort of thing off.

And, oh boy, did Rosie start to get ballsy as time went by and she felt comfortable enough to come out of her shell, not that she was ever really in her shell to begin with! About a year into my job at the site, I remember the shenanigans that went on at the annual staff Christmas party. Rosie had turned up to the event wearing rather tight, white, very slightly see-through pants—with no underwear, I take it, at least from the comments being made! Some of the men were enjoying her squeezing past them to get to her seat.

Anyway, after much singing and even dancing from the group, I remember how Rosie stood up to sing a personal number to Edward's boss, James Hardy. The words were strung together in a silly but amusing way and involved pointing out her value to the site. At one point, she talked about how she had more balls than all the men in the room combined, although I have to say she had a point there! And at the end of each verse, she threw in a reminder to James Hardy that he should give her a pay raise.

By the end of the night, after a few drinks, Rosie had appointed herself event photographer and was in the men's bathroom taking photos of the guys as they visited the urinals. I'm not sure if all the urinal photos were posted, but I saw at least four or five photos of guys' butts on the Valcorp intranet the next day. I'm rather surprised no one complained, actually! But it was a laid-back group. Secretly, I thought it was all hilarious, but shh. I don't want to admit to being politically incorrect.

However, despite the huge amount of entertainment I was getting from her antics, I could also feel how the pressure and stress at the site was building up over time. Rosie was making it her business to challenge everyone who stood up to her in any way. One day, when a trainer came out from Germany to commission a new extrusion machine we'd put in, I watched with shock as Rosie was rude and made fun of the man in front of the operating staff.

He was a technical man, and I think he was giving explanations that were over her head. I commented that I understood and his training was useful. "Please go on." But Rosie went to great lengths to ask him questions about site-specific problems and laugh at him and correct him when his answers weren't in line with hers. She made him look like a joke in front of operators, who weren't technical enough to understand what was being said, and I thought, what a waste of a training opportunity. Why bully a man who's doing his best to help you here?

Later in time, that was the way she would begin to talk to me when I, too, talked about technical things that were over her head. She would make combative, incorrect comments designed to make me look like I was the stupid one in front of a confused audience.

Another day, probably about two years into my time in the job, a temporary manager, Felix, came in to replace Edward while he spent some months overseas scouting out new product opportunities. I hadn't even met Felix yet when Tony pulled me aside to chat to me about what had gone on in his introduction meeting with Felix. Apparently, Felix had asked Tony seriously, "Do you think Michelle is intelligent enough to actually do the job, or do you think we need to be looking for someone more competent for the position?"

Tony had been taken aback and had replied that I was highly intelligent and capable, of which Felix seemed unconvinced and explained that Rosie didn't seem to think so. Before I had even met him! Rosie had gotten in his ear to convince him that I ought to be replaced!

In the midst of all this, Hugo was also adding pressure out on the floor by creating competition between the staff. One of his new performance initiatives was to divide the shifts into three colors and pit them against each other. One of Valcorp's core values, after all, was "A sense of urgency," so I suppose he was achieving exactly what the company desired. But boy, could you feel the tension.

The ladies who were packing the cups were starting to have serious arguments over whether the previous shift had laid out enough boxes for the next, and who could claim the box of cups produced during the changeover. Heaven forbid anyone make a lot of scrap! One day, there was quite an upset when a larger lady pushed down a smaller, heavily pregnant lady while arguing during changeover.

I started to become uncomfortable about asking for help with trial preparations or changes I needed made when everyone was so busy focused on rapid production and not losing any time. My Aspie self was definitely not a fan of having to press other people to get things done, and I started to avoid the tasks where I needed other people's help, even if it meant doing more strenuous work myself or tasks taking longer.

One day, after only several months working at the site, I was told to come in late as there was an important operator-only meeting to be called in the morning. By the time I came in, 25 percent of the staff had been made redundant (fired). The way it was put to me was that they were the ones with "bad attitudes," although I know it really translated to the ones that Rosie didn't like any more. The turnover at the site was crazy!

And in the stress of it all, I found myself starting to suffer again from that work-place sick-in-the-stomach feeling that I'd had at all my other jobs. This time, it was more confusing for me to be sure where it was coming from, because there were so many possible causes. Was it due to all complicated politics and the pressure I had to work under, or was it just the same old thing all over again—a problem with me?

When it got too much for me, every now and then, I would go sit in the bathroom for ten to twenty minutes until the nausea went down. I couldn't really stay in there any longer than that without it being a problem.

I also found sanctuary in sitting briefly in between rows of sheet rolls in the ware-house. The warehouse was quiet and dimly lit and felt so calming in comparison to all the bright lights of the factory. Being between the rows of product and resin all neatly lined up strangely uplifted me. Such order. It was very satisfying. But I couldn't stay in there too long either, lest I be missed. Most days, all I could think about was how I just wanted to get out of there!

To add mayhem to madness, I also started to have some awkward interactions with Tony while going about our day-to-day business. For a long time, Tony and I got along exceptionally well. Just like I had in high school, he was my one-on-one friend whom I wanted to spend all my time talking to. We spent many hours completing tests in the laboratory with just the two of us discussing work and the people at our work. We went out for long lunches, just one-on-one. He was one of the best friends I'd ever had.

Somewhere along the track, however, Tony decided that he had developed feel-ings for me, which was somewhat uncomfortable, as I never saw him that way. I was married. He was married. It wasn't a case of him losing interest in his wife. It was always clear that he loved her dearly. But he'd started thinking things about me too and just wanted me to know about it. He was a lot older than I was, and I made it clear that it was not mutual. In turn, he was careful to make sure I knew that I could say no and I would not jeopardize my work in any way, shape, or form. He just wanted things to be known and out on the table, whatever the outcome.

I often think back to myself and wonder if Tony actually did anything wrong in this. I know that the law would say yes. It is sexual harassment. But don't we all have inappropriate thoughts about others from time to time? I guess, then, we might con-clude that the line should be drawn such that it's okay to have thoughts but not okay to tell others about them.

But what if you're like Tony and have a compulsion to be completely open and honest with others at all times? Everything about Tony screams complete honesty in communication. I can understand this. I'm very much that way inclined myself. Tony was always respectful and polite, and I never felt pressured to go along with it. The rules of "morals" are really only constructs created by society. They don't always apply to every case. I'm still undecided on the issue.

Tony enjoyed my company and started being everywhere I went. I enjoyed the companionship and support. He would run his trials and do his share of the work and then come back in to be around for mine as well. It was never really a problem except for the impressions it gave other people, which I came to understand much later on.

Over time, unfortunately, Tony felt the need to sporadically check if my feelings had changed in any way. The answer was always the same: they had not. It started to make me uncomfortable, having the topic broached over and over again. I tried to be okay with it for his sake, because he was such a positive friend for me, but eventually, I couldn't.

After I left Valcorp some time later, I didn't contact Tony for the first few years. It had built up to a point that was too awkward for me to handle. It was such a waste of a unique friendship. Only recently, I've started having email contact with Tony again, and maybe with time, I'll even find a way to be comfortable with him in person and we can recommence as friends. But baby steps. I don't think he would make the same mistake again.

Sigh. It seems life is definitely not black and white the way we're taught in story books growing up. It's complicated and grey. At this time in my life, I was feeling confused about a lot of things.

To be continued . . .

Chapter Twenty-Four

Asperger's Syndrome and Bullying

I remember, toward the end of my time at Valcorp Ringwood, having a thought once about why bullying types like to target me so much. It just seemed to be becoming a pattern, and I couldn't figure out, why me? Had it happened only during high school, I could've dismissed it as bad luck or due to an unfortunate rumor. But when I find myself in the same position again in adulthood, the question starts to become puzzling. I really don't see how I'm attracting the negative attention.

My first thought about it was, am I bringing it upon myself in any way? I've heard discussions before about some people having a "victim's mentality" that can draw bullies or abusers toward them. I considered that, in high school, it's possible that this could've been the case. I had a lower self-esteem back then. However, in adulthood, I've learnt to carry myself with confidence and am well able to hold my own in a discussion or debate. I no longer give the appearance of "weakness," nor am I someone who's particularly subject to peer pressure or coercion.

Actually, to be honest, I'm probably a little *too* resistant to it and ignore the group entirely if what they're up to doesn't align with my goals. And I am the least likely type to be guilt-tripped into anything or feel compelled to act as a doormat. Conform? Who, me? I doubt it. So what is it about me, I wondered, that could possibly be attracting these types?

Then one day, I had a realization that made lot of sense. This isn't happening because of anything I'm doing wrong. I'm not specifically seeking out or attracting the attention. Bullies just like to target people like me because I am different and *alone* in comparison to the rest of the group.

To use a strange analogy to illustrate my point, which is a very "me" way to describe it, imagine for a second a pack of wild deer being hunted. The predators that come in will probably pick on the weak and injured if they get a chance, but that isn't their primary target. Even more appealing is that deer that is off to the side, the one that has wandered that bit too far and is separated from the herd. It makes for an easy attack and kill, as, after all, a one-on-one fight is so much easier than having to contend with the whole herd.

In human society, it occurs to me that I am that deer, the one without the network of friends that would come running to my defense. Attacking me doesn't cause damage to a person's social standing, as I'm never really in any social groups anyway. It makes me the perfect, low-risk target. So I suppose it wouldn't matter what I did—I may always draw some of that sort of attention.

In my wonderings about the topic, I also realized that I could be an easy target for repeat bullying simply because I'm not aggressive or too inclined to fight back. During my high school years, when various acts of bullying were going on, I never actually told anybody about it—not the teachers, nor parents, nor peers. No one. I know it seems crazy now, but at the time, it just never occurred to me. My logical mind went about trying to comprehend this problem as it did all others: quietly, on my own. And in hindsight, I can see that telling a teacher may have been a helpful and sensible thing to do. But to a sixteen-year-old me, that wasn't obvious.

I also think that perhaps I found it harder than my fellow students to even be sure what those behaviors were. I'd never encountered indirect aggression before, and sometimes, it was tricky for me to distinguish something as bullying behavior as opposed to just confusing typical behavior.

For example, in senior school, there was one girl in my class who used to occasionally grab me and spin me around just for fun. It didn't hurt me, so it didn't really bother me that she did that. In fact, I liked the attention and thought that perhaps it was a friendly gesture, despite the fact that she did it in a pushy way. Much later in my adult life, I came to understand what she was doing. She was signaling to the other girls in the room, "Look, everyone. I can make Michelle do whatever I want, so I'm better than her." A status play.

I guess Aspies don't naturally think about or fight for status, so I never recognized the behavior as somewhat degrading. It makes me wonder, actually, how many other degrading behaviors I've allowed because I didn't really think anything of them.

Looking back on my Valcorp Ringwood experience, I also see now that had I been out and about talking to people and promoting myself, then it wouldn't have been so easy for colleagues to sabotage my work or use me as a scapegoat. Social schmoozing was the game that everyone else was playing, yet there I was keeping mostly to myself and talking directly only to my boss, Tony. I'd made myself that lone deer again, way off in the far foliage.

Of course, I'm not and have never been the social butterfly or schmoozing type, and I doubt I ever will be. And that's okay. I am the way I am. But I have to be aware that it does make me vulnerable in the wrong sort of environment.

Now, wandering back to the goings-on in my teenage years, I made a point one day to sit down and write a few words to a teen being bullied that I would have liked to have heard at the time. And I would like to include those words here, because I think they form some important understanding all teenagers should have.

So here's my little flyer on it:

> **Bullying**
>
> People do not target you because there is anything wrong with **you**.
>
> They target you because there is something missing in **them**.
>
> The types of people who enjoy putting others down—directly or covertly—do it because without it, they do not feel good/strong/ important enough within themselves. Abusing others gives a temporary high. It makes the person bullying feel clever or funny or tough or better than the person they are mistreating. But the feeling only lasts so long before they start to feel ordinary again and need another "hit" (not unlike a drug addiction). Remember that normal, healthy people do not go around trying to put others down. Repetitive bullying behavior is a sign of a troubled person and should always be reported to a trusted adult.

Now, correct me if I'm on my own little tangent here, but I thought that text like this might help teens, because it doesn't just say "don't bully." It calls it out for the weakness that it actually is. I thought if bullying were understood this way, perhaps it wouldn't seem like such a cool thing for peers and the other students around to imitate. Perhaps it would no longer seem cool at all, and that's what I would hope to achieve.

So I just wanted to put that out there.

But anyway, that's enough attempts to fix the world for one chapter. Moving on . . .

Having written most of this chapter about bullying and the reasons behind it, I keep being reminded, actually, of a girl in my high school, Nadia, whom I mentioned once before. In early Year Ten, she was a main perpetrator of my teasing. She was so quick with words—even to the point of being talented—and would always be on the ball with a comment to make in the form of a little dig here or there. There was just something about her sharp, cutting, subtle edge that the other girls thought was hilarious, and sometimes, others would emulate her and try and join in on her popularity that way. So it sort of created a little mob that would taunt me every now and then.

Then, over a few months, she stopped. Just like that. It was odd. In that short time, she even started acting friendly and chatted to me on occasion and asked me questions about myself, with nothing negative to say in reply. What was the catch, I wondered.

One day, in a conversation later on, she mentioned to me that she'd been going to anger management counseling. Perhaps it was an apology of sorts, or at least an explanation. At the time, it sounded strange to me, because she didn't strike me as an angry person. She seemed witty and popular. But what I didn't yet understand was that anger and frustration, as emotions, aren't always expressed directly. The "anger issues" she referred to had been the cause of her subtle spite in wit, and once she began dealing with those core issues, she didn't feel the need to be like that anymore.

It's a funny thing how anger can manifest itself in so many subtle and different ways and a worrying thing I never really understood any of that until so much later in my life. Now that I'm an adult and have made sense of the nature of unkind and taunting behaviors, I'm much more protected from it than I ever used to be. But in the meanwhile, I hope there will be others to look out for, stick up for, and guide all the other Aspie teens and young adults out there who may be in the same position—confused, alone, and/or not knowing what to do about it—as I once was. Because, as Aspies, really, how are we supposed to have a clue?

CHAPTER TWENTY-FIVE

DO ASPIES LIE?

Q: Do Aspies lie?

Ummm . . . Well, that's an unusual question, and I guess I have a simple answer for this: No, not really. Not if we can avoid it. Most of the Aspies I know find lying, deception, or inaccuracy of any kind to be uncomfortable and unnatural for us. We have a natural urge to correct things and want to make them accurate and properly representative. So purposely saying something that's false goes against the grain.

Of course, like any group in society, there will always be some individuals who don't fit the mold. I've heard of Aspies who regularly lie. In fact, I've even heard of Aspies (from online posts at least) who have become excellent at lying and take pride in how well they're able to deceive others. To me, this seems so against the Aspie way of thinking that I almost wonder if it comes from a misdiagnosis of sociopathy, borderline personality disorder, or some other condition. Either way, I'm sure that Aspies of this sort are rare.

But for most of us, lying is only something we do under compelling circumstances or when made clear that to lie is the social expectation, and even then, it doesn't always sit right with us. I know many Aspies find the social standard of telling "white lies" to be distasteful. If someone says to me, "Do you like my new haircut?" and I don't, it's inconceivable to me to say, "Yes, that looks gorgeous on you!"

It's a direct lie, and I can't do it, yet I know that to lie is the neurotypical expec-tation in these circumstances, and to fail to tell a white lie would be offensive. So I've learned to compromise by avoiding the question and focusing on something positive, such as, "Oh, wow, those color streaks look really interesting!" (Even though the cut is unflattering and your hair now highlights the rolls under your chin!)

In a way, it seems silly to me that people ask questions that they don't really want to hear the true answer to, but I suppose it's all part of that social bonding and showing support to your friends that people like to do.

I still get myself in trouble sometimes for being too blunt with the truth. I guess it's because my concern in answering a question is usually on giving the right answer, not on what others want me to say or whether my reply could make the other person feel negative in any way. The concept that there even is an alternative answer to the true one feels a bit twisted and wrong to me.

I think this sort of bluntness in Aspies is a common trait, and we all get feedback from time to time that we're too blunt or rude to varying degrees. Of course, some of us have a better handle on the rules of what to say and how to say it than others, and this is something we do learn with time and experience.

Chapter Twenty-Six

Asperger's and Imagination

Q: I've heard people say that Autistics can often have vivid imaginations and are known to sometimes retreat into fantasy worlds. Is this true?

Oh, good. Now I get to move on to a fun topic!

I think a rather vivid imagination is a trait that many Autistics and Aspies share to varying degrees. In a discussion with the League some months back, I remember one fellow Aspie, Rob, sharing how he liked to take journeys into outer space. He described the fantasy as being so real, he could feel the sun on his back.

Another man, David N., explained how when he feels life is hard and his anxiety is heightened, he struggles not to withdraw into his own world. He talked about getting images, such as people stabbing at his head, as an expression of his emotions. I can imagine Aspies in general being prone to escapism in any form that encourages retreat into visual fantasy; e.g., role-playing games, reading, anime, etc. We seem to have an extra ability to really feel and engage in these images.

I know that, for me, I find reading hard to snap out of. If I particularly like a book, I'll read it cover to cover and avoid stopping even to eat, sleep, do housework, or do any other thing I ought to be doing. Any interruption agitates me, and I rush through what I need to do to get back to the story. I never fully disengage.

After completing a book, I can then find myself stuck in the emotions at the end of the book for days on end, unable to snap out of the mood or stop thinking about the storyline. It causes me a lot of trouble when I read books with melancholy or flat endings. I also found role-playing games in my teen years to be similarly consuming. Fortunately, I don't read or play these games that often or I think I would become an emotional wreck!

And while I'm not so heavily engaged in visual fantasies as some of my Aspie peers, I do have a tendency to be visual when it comes to imagining or recalling scenery and places I like. One day in Houston, when feeling homesick, I made this post on Facebook about missing home. (I'll explain how I ended up in Houston a little later on in the book.)

"I wish I could walk down a path on the beach and find an isolated beach area all to myself and sit on the rocks and listen to the waves crash against the rocks. And Isaac could play in the little rock pools and find strange and interesting creatures and boulders . . .

"I wish I could go to a wildlife walk and have the whole place to myself and sit and listen to the birds and animals and wind blowing in the trees . . .

"I wish I could go down my parents' yard and walk along fallen trees to the creek or lay in the soft grass (not like Houston grass!!) and watch the trees swaying and the clouds moving along the sky until it almost feels like I'm moving and not the clouds. And just relax and recharge and be happy, with not a person or building in sight."

Each scene I was visualizing in striking detail, far more details than I was able to describe in a brief online post.

Another evening, after wandering some parkland with my camera, I remember jotting down these notes on the visions that the walk inspired in me. I often have similar visions of nature and imagery. They're such a soothing thing to just relax and dwell upon.

Now my editor has told me that this next section gets a bit boring and I should consider cutting some of it out, but I decided to ignore that advice, because I think it's a good example of just how much detail the Aspie mind goes into. So shhh, don't tell her I left it in! We can just nod and agree and pretend it's gone. *wink wink*[33] But if you do happen to get bored as you read down, please feel free to skip forward to the last paragraph of the quote!

"After a glorious day's walk in the park with my camera, I come home and find my mind full of visions of foliage. Every time I shut my eyes, there is a new image, crisp and clear and vivid in its detail. You would think they would be of the plants I've seen during the day, but they seem to be new visions I've never seen before, each one stunning and radiating color. Perfect in every detail. Symmetrical, with no messy parts. Like the perfect photography shot.

---

[33] Editor's note: I see what you did there, Michelle! ;-)

"I see a tuft of sturdy grass like stems poking out of the water. The tuft is creating ripples outward as if agitated by the wind. The dark green of the tuft is highlighted against the nearly black water. Of course, the water might be clearer if it were real life, but in this lighting, the hue of the water appears particularly dark against the light of the grass and sky. The image shows only the one central tuft and is crisp and free of other reflections or messiness that would crowd the frame. The black ripples come and go in little gusts.

"I see a tree branch coated in yellowish, even slightly off-green moss. I can make out the detail in the moss pattern. The branch itself has creamy white/grey bark with little spirals of bark pattern in the visible patches between the moss. Far off in the background, I see a blur of green bracken. The bracken itself is perfect in its evenness, each frond growing to exactly the same height.

"I see a zoomed-in shot of a new leaf budding out of a cut-off stump of wood. Just a thin, clean, pale, pine-colored cut. You can sort of make out the circles in the wood. The leaf itself is uncurling, a little like a fern frond, but thicker and furry. Its pale green stands out and complements the stump. I can see the detail of the fur on the edges of each leaf.

"I see purple flowers wilting off the end of long green stems. They're small and wispy. The flowers, not perfectly crisp, hang downward in a trumpet shape, delicate and thin like lightly crinkled paper. The crinkles are uniform and visually appealing. Each flower hangs off a single stem, displaying an array of aligned green stems. The pale purple/lilac makes a nice contrast against the light, slightly yellowed green. The background is a similar, darker green blur of clover and teardrop-shaped leaves, although to me, they are not the center of focus and hard to make out individually.

"I see a flower in a shape almost too odd to describe. It has a circular center with a long protruding stem. Its 'petals,' if you call them that, reach outward like elongated fingers. The whole thing is red/green, not in crisp sections of color but mottled red/green color gradients. Its shape is distinctive and perfectly formed. It gives me the impression of some exotic species that targets flies and insects or even moves its fingers to entrap them upon touch.

"Some of the images aren't even in real-life colors. It's like a picture that has been edited. I see a plant in a vivid yellow-green glow. A series of leaves radiate outward from a central vein. It's patterned like a fern, but with thicker, crisper leaves of defined shape. Each one is an elongated rectangle rounded into a curve at the end. In perfect series, they transition from larger to smaller. The whole leaf is not visible, as if it's been cropped. The radiating yellow/green is striking.

"I wish I could put my camera into my head to capture them. They're magnificent, image after image after image, each as stunning and detailed as the next. I wonder where my mind draws them from and how it keeps generating them."

Sometimes, when I'm feeling particularly positive about who I am, or occasionally as an attempt to cheer myself up, I focus on this image I have of myself standing in a grassy area, which is actually the front lawn of a library back at home.

There are a few trees around me, and on that particular day, the colors are radiant. The bright green of new grass encapsulates me. I'm standing in the center of the grass with my arms stretched out, spinning in the sunlight. Of course, I never really stood there and spun in real life as I know that would be strange, but it was something I imagined doing, walking past the scene one day. My hair is shining golden in the sun. It does that. The feeling of letting my hair flow in the wind makes me feel light and free.

In this image, all the beauty and magnanimity on the inside is radiating outward. It is just an image, and I don't know why it has this effect, but it reminds me of who I am and what I stand for. It's about beauty and love and peace and caring for others and seeing the good in people. It's me.

So I suppose I do share some components of that common Aspie vivid imagination, and I have to say, I love it. The images I create are inspiring and relaxing and help me feel at peace with the world. I've read suggestions before that Aspies are so inclined toward fantasy and retreat because they want to escape from the overstimulation and stress of the real world, and I can see how escapism could be tempting. But I myself am pretty tuned into life around me and don't have a problem with "fading out," so I see no negatives in it.

I see such images more as something to enjoy in a world that's often hectic and unpleasant otherwise. They're inspiration to go out and do and create beautiful things. It maintains my feelings of peace, joy, and purpose in an otherwise flat sort of existence. To have passion makes life. To have no passion feels dead inside. I'm glad I have this ability to fantasize.

CHAPTER TWENTY-SEVEN

VALCORP RINGWOOD—PART TWO

So, going back into my little world at Valcorp Ringwood . . .

At this point in time, as my workplace started to feel like a psychological mine-field, I was also starting to discover a few upsides to this little company that made it so difficult to walk away. With the money rolling in from new customers and jobs, Edward started to tease us with a taste of the high life. We were taken out to expensive restaurants like the Waterfront at the Crown Casino in Melbourne and a private dining floor booked for us at the Flower Drum, which I hear has a price tag of over $200 a head! It certainly filled us with feelings of grandeur and importance.

One day, I remember taking a taxi in with Tony to the Crown Casino, all dressed up in a long, black evening gown with a slit down one side up to my thigh. The front of the dress was cut into a V shape that dipped a little below my breasts, with jewels hanging down from the middle and with high heels on my legs, which looked like they went on forever. On the elevator on the way to the restaurant, Tony amused me by pointing out the looks he was getting from other people. "They must think I'm rich," he explained to me—older man, attractive young woman, both dressed up in elaborate attire. He couldn't wipe the grin off his face.

Back at the site, Tony and I also had a lot of comical moments joking around with the guys and the ladies on the factory floor. One day, I just about fell over from laughter when I came down to find Tony with a large, black stripe extending into one side of his mouth and out of the other. He was completely unaware of it. Apparently, he'd marked and cut out some plastic to do a test on the sheet properties while out on the line and had held his marked sample in his mouth while setting up his machine, hence the permanent marker clown mouth.

When I told Tony, he had a little chuckle and decided to leave it there while he finished up his work. He chatted to a few operators and let them get a kick out of it too. He was very comfortable with himself like that and didn't see the need to put on a formal air.

One week, I even went through the training course to get a forklift license. Yes, me, Ms. Clumsy who trips over and walks into everything! When I sat the test, I remember how a crowd of guys from the factory floor had stood around watching and were almost falling over with laughter every time I accidentally jerked the forklift controls or reversed instead of going forward. But with cheers of encouragement, I passed the test and was given a license to drive and learn the forklift further. Hooray for me!

In between all the fun out on the line, however, the day shifts in the office were becoming increasingly high pressure, as I mentioned before. Edward wanted everyone to work long hours to keep up with the new projects that needed to move forward. He frequently used his line about staff giving 110 percent and drew charts on the whiteboard to illustrate his point.

One day, I worked on trials for more than twenty-four hours in a row before an operator, Allen, came in to relieve me of the role. I was really supposed to stay until all the trials were finished, but kindly, Allen insisted I couldn't work any longer and he could handle it. Unfortunately, although he worked hard, the sheet trial that time failed, and they couldn't get the product in specification. I don't think Edward or Hugo were too impressed the trial needed to be re-run.

On another occasion, I insisted—well in advance—that I wasn't going to be available on a particular day, as it was my father-in-law's 60th birthday celebration. As the day approached, the trial of course fell on that day, and I put my foot down and said sorry, but I wouldn't be coming in. It caused the production schedule to be interrupted, and Edward had a word to me about how disappointed he was, telling me lines like, "You don't help yourself, Michelle." He told me he was worried that my commitment to the job wasn't strong enough, notably because of something he was sensing about my demeanor.

I think what he was picking up on was really my reluctance to do some parts of the job, like calling around or approaching contractors and unfamiliar people. It was my Aspie exhaustion talking. But, of course, Edward translated it as lack of motivation or proper dedication. He said he didn't think I was giving 110 percent.

Sometimes, Edward tried to help me by giving me tips on how to interact with people. "Don't tell them everything you know right away," I remember him advising me. "Hold on to some of it. Use it to your advantage."

He wanted me to be more politically savvy and come across as more cool and powerful, but I guess I just wasn't getting it. I have a way of coming across as me, not as one of the cool clique. I'm more just someone who is always off in my own little world doing my own little thing and then trying eagerly to join in the moment I think of something I want to say. I can't really be anything else, and slowly, I could see that I was losing Edward's backing.

And the arguments in the management office were getting fierce. I remember one day, toward the end of my time at the plant, how I'd attended a staffing meeting in Tony's absence. A relatively new supervisor, Neal, had been recruited all the way from America after Rosie and Edward had run an expensive international recruitment campaign to find experienced operators.

Neal always had a soft and gentle manner, which had pleased Rosie at first. He believed in empowering people and building teams rather than the kick-butt methods usually employed at Valcorp. Some of the operators were not used to his style and made fun of his soft approach. They imitated the little one-liners he used to say, such as, "Donkeys look at each other and kick the problem. Hyenas look at the problem and kick each other," thinking it was funny and missing the reason that he came up with such lines. However, all was going at least okay for him until he started to stand firm against Rosie interfering with his shift and his management style.

Very quickly, Rosie went from being happy with Neal to whispering in Edward's and Hugo's ears about his incompetence.

Anyway, long story short, in that meeting, the group had a discussion on what should be done about Neal's difficulties as a supervisor. Hugo started to talk about the possibility of training or coaching him, to which Rosie brashly interrupted something along the lines of, "Forget that. I'm going to watch him until he does something wrong and get the bugger fired."

Shortly after, Neal was issued a warning letter for some mistake he'd made out on the line. It's the standard protocol for fair dismissal in Australia for a person to receive at least a warning letter first about actions that need improving. A week or two later, he quit, under further pressure, I'm sure. I'm guessing it better to quit and move on than be fired and have to explain it to the next employer.

I was rather shocked by how rapidly Neal departed. It seemed like one minute there was a problem, and the next, I blinked and he was gone! After that, things started to go downhill rapidly for me as well in the same manner.

Come pay raise time at the plant, I had a moment where I remember opening my pay slip and being shocked to read that I would be receiving no bonus that year and a pay rise only in line with inflation. At Valcorp, annual bonuses were standard, and I'd considered a bonus of around $5,000 to be part of my salary package. Tony had given me an excellent performance review and had written many positive things about me, so I wasn't expecting what felt like a pay cut.

I marched upstairs—not angrily, just assertively—to ask Edward why my bonus and pay rise had been so low, to which he flatly told me he didn't think I added any value to the business. What a line to hear! "You don't add any value to the business." He commented that I'm always in training and don't do a lot of work on my own. "Training," I came understand, was how Tony had been justifying his extra time with me on paper. As Tony was the only person who ever actually saw my work, Edward had decided, quite bluntly, that it wasn't all that valuable.

In the moment, it stunned me, because I'd been working hard to see that plant grow and succeed. I spent a great deal of time on the line every day checking and double checking to make everything always run smoothly—always without being asked. That was my commitment.

Very coolly, I sort of frowned at Edward and threw a comment back about there perhaps being other reasons that Tony was around me all the time. In hindsight, it wasn't the best thing to say, but I guess defensiveness got the better of me in the moment.

The next day, I came to work to find Tony upset. It seems Edward had gone straight to Tony the previous night to tell him how I'd tried to "backstab" him and "throw him under the bus" by making insinuations. Tony wasn't mad at me but insisted that he was upset at how much trouble him being around me had caused for my salary and reputation. He also had admitted he was hurt by how it had all gone down, but again made clear that he wasn't mad at me. He understood.

Argh. I was so mad at Edward for handling it that way. What a mess.

Sometime after that, Edward pulled me upstairs to talk about my phone records. He told me how he'd had me researched by the company to see who I had been contacting and look into how often I called Tony. However, instead of me calling Tony a lot, he'd found a lot of texts between me and an operator at the plant. He said it with a grin like he'd found something interesting. I shrugged it off—it was banter. But it did leave me wondering just how much he'd dug into to investigate me. It was a strange invasion of privacy.

All the while, I'd been getting increasingly depressed and stressed just from that awful feeling of just needing to get away from the workplace. Some days, I think I enjoyed the high of attention from one of the operators to get me through the days. It's not something I would ever lock onto now, but sometimes, attention can be like a drug.

It's the high of escapism, and I was looking for anything to grab onto to keep myself together!

At this point, you may ask why I didn't just quit the job. What on Earth would possess me to stay in such a toxic environment? But you see, I was starting to see a pattern. It wasn't just in this job that I was having trouble. It was in all of them.

As much as I didn't want it to be true, this is what I kept finding:

- Every place I worked, I had an overwhelming desire to get out of there.

- I had trouble focusing on the work and interacting with people at the same time. I would feel frustrated or angry inside and often felt like snapping at people (although I didn't).

- I dreaded having to do tasks that involved dealing with unfamiliar people. It exhausted me.

- I disliked having to figure out how to do new things. Most of the time, I was given new things constantly, and I really had to force myself to start them.

- I had trouble remembering verbal instructions and needed to write things down.

- I often felt as if other people were technically incompetent.

- In hindsight, perhaps I didn't do and say the right things to project the best image of myself and promote myself to others.

- I needed to do things my way and plan my own time. Being micromanaged by others was too stressful.

- I felt sick and started to hate going to work.

All I could conclude was that the common factor was me. I didn't know why, but I was the problem. So what would be the point of starting over somewhere new when I would just have to go through it all over again? Besides, I loved this little Ringwood plant, if only I could work there without all the management staff. (And turn the lights off too!)

By this point, strong feelings of uselessness had crept into my head. I didn't think I could ever start a new job and do any better. I just didn't have the energy to try again. I'd resigned to just try and cope if I could.

In hindsight, I wish I could go back in time and teach myself how to separate the weaknesses I perceived in myself from unfair treatment. I would explain to myself that no matter how bad at politics I am, I still deserve to be treated kindly and with respect. I would point out that while I have weaknesses, I also have strengths—valuable strengths. And a good company should nurture a person's talents and help them find ways to work around their weaknesses.

Not being strong in every area doesn't make you a failure. It took me time to come to these realizations—many years, in fact. At the time of this story, I was far too trapped in confusion and depressed emotions to see the picture clearly.

Anyway, one evening, when I was particularly alone and despondent and just couldn't handle the idea of going into work one more day, I did something awful and hurt myself. Even writing that, I'm ashamed and want to scratch it from my writing, but I need to say it, as it's an important part of the story.

It would be easy to just dismiss it as an act of stupidity or something thoughtless and impulsive, but the truth is, when you're drowning in that much emotion, it's not something you do as an accident. It's a logical thing—anything to make the pain go away. For me, it was also anything to escape work the next day and the next and the next. When I woke up the next morning, it did feel like a stupid thing to have done, and I hid it away for a while.

When I came back to work the next week, I remember Tony was still talking about my pay issues and how annoyed he was that Edward had passed on my pay rise without even consulting him. I was his staff, and he thought that was just downright disrespectful.

I'd taken a day off work on the Monday after "the incident"—which I will call it, as anything else just sounds too embarrassing to say out loud—and that Tuesday, I was feeling somber and not at all in the mood to discuss the pay raise issue or what I'd done. So I just pressed on with my day. But after a few days at work, I did manage to bring "the incident" up. Just to Tony. I don't think I could have told anyone else.

As you can imagine, Tony was mortified and admitted he had had some idea something was wrong. I can't remember his immediate reaction, as I'd sort of felt awkward and looked away. It's times like these where I especially can't look at people.

But I remember shortly afterward, in a fired-up state, he strode on up to Edward and Felix and had a serious talk with them. (Felix was the temporary manager I mentioned earlier who'd taken over while Edward was scouting for marketing opportunities overseas. At this point, he hadn't yet handed the plant back to Edward.) Tony was extremely emotional and red-hot motivated to get things back to the way they used to be. Perhaps he was hoping I'd be compensated too for all the stress I'd been put through.

After a little time for deliberation, I remember Edward called a private meeting with me, just one-on-one. We sat in an empty room together, and he reached out to me and let me know that I could get assistance from the company if I wanted counseling or the like. His manner was comforting. However, he did impress upon me—just between me and him, person to person—that if I did report the incident, the whole of Valcorp upper management would need to know about it and they would probably not take me as seriously in the future. It could impact my future pay rises or ability to get promoted within the company.

I was starting to feel ashamed about the whole thing and reluctantly agreed not to report it. I put it aside in my head and conceded to let it slide. In turn, Felix, as temporary manager, allowed me part-time work to take some of the pressure off me, which I was very thankful for. I needed that relief of the odd day off!

I would like to say it all settled in well from there and working part time was the break I needed, but unfortunately, when Edward moved back into the role as plant manager, he decided he had other plans for me. He moved me upstairs into my own office, where I was no longer privy to any plant conversations, and told me I would report directly to him from then on.

But then he never did come into my office to give me any work to do or pass on information about the goings-on in the plant. Sometimes, operators or other staff were sent out onto the factory floor to do parts of my job without telling me, which was exasperating to me as I didn't know what was going on with the equipment. When I asked about work, Edward assigned me a different task—database design work—and told me that was my top priority and I should focus on that. It required communicating with others and waiting for them to get back to me—not work that I enjoyed!—and really only took up an hour or two in the day at most.

One afternoon, tired of not knowing what to do, I caught him down in the management office and insisted that I was short on work and needed more to do, but his response embarrassed me. He—without yelling—berated me publically, exclaiming, "Look around at how busy everyone else is. There is an excess of work to be done. Take some initiative!" But how could I when I had no idea what was happening in the plant around me? I was out of that all-important information loop. I didn't try to ask him for work again but instead retreated to the office and tried to find ways to while away the extra time.

Within just a week or two of him being back in charge, he informed me of some "good news." He'd organized for me to transfer to Mooroopna, a site four hours' drive north of where I lived, to do further database design work, which I could do on a part-time basis.

The whole offer infuriated me. I'd only just gotten back to living where I had friends and family around and was determined not to be torn away and lonely again. When I indicated that I didn't want to move out to Mooroopna and didn't accept the transfer, he looked at me coolly and said, "Well, I don't see a place for you in the future of this plant." I understood it as a threat that I would have to go one way or another.

Now, I know that I could've fought on and stayed in my role regardless, but at this point, I decided there was just no gain in it. I didn't want to be the person I would have to become to survive at this site any more. It was either I change—become aggressive and fight my way back in—or leave. And so, the next morning, I handed my resignation letter to Edward, which he looked a little too pleased to receive. I think he felt he had victory. How easily he'd won over me.

Edward announced my resignation to the entire team in the management meeting that morning. The speed with which he did it and lack of deliberation on his part really confirmed his stance on having me there. He had me verbally fill out an exit form—which he insisted he would do the writing for—and then had me sign it. I didn't make it hard for him. I told the truth but kept it brief and left off the details so I could leave in an impartial way. After all, burning my bridges wasn't likely to be helpful. And then by the end of the week, I'd handed over my things and left.

What a relief to not have to go in anymore! What a socially confusing situation, to now be without a job and really not want to seek another one. It left me floating for a while, taking time for the numbness that had been my life at Valcorp to wear off and for me to slowly find myself again. To feel again.

The good news is that this is the worst chapter in my story, and it only goes up from there. So you can breathe a sigh of relief now! It's over. It's over! Oh, thank God it's over. I never want to go through an experience like that again.

The week after I left, Tony, who'd been outraged by their whole way of handling me, followed and resigned as well. I sort of always knew he would. He said that he could no longer work for a company that he didn't respect or want to support. So in the end, their whole technical team walked out in a matter of days, which was a little amusing to me.

Edward tried to compel Tony to come back by offering him more money. He even said Tony could have two new staff to replace me if he wanted, which only insulted Tony more and cemented his decision. At some point, Edward said to Tony something along the lines of, "I'm screwed, aren't I?" And that was the last I ever heard of Edward. Rosie, I hear, got a promotion into marketing but was fired not long after, because apparently, the new site didn't enjoy her attitude as much as Edward had. I have no idea where she works now.

Not to brag or be vindictive, but I can't resist mentioning that after we left the plant, I heard feedback about the plant having serious problems with scraps due to errors in production and setup. Management, of course, attributed it to "operator incompetence" and gave warnings to the team leaders. But you can't expect operators to foresee everything when you have shifts changing in and out and new products coming and going. You need a person to coordinate it all and be in charge of communication. That person was me.

The site produced thousands of dollars of scrap over many runs during the next few months. They also got an expert in to assess some of the problems in sheet quality who told them that the cooling rollers needed replacing. Surprise, surprise. I'd been telling them that for the last year but had been argued down.

I know that Edward must've realized in the week that followed that he'd made a mistake in driving me to leave. Sometimes, staff are not a dime a dozen. Some staff are hard to replace. Chewing them up and spitting them out can come back to bite you! But I'm not one to interfere or follow up on the situation. I just check in every now and then with my sources here and there and grin when I hear what disaster has gone on next. I know that's bad, but can you blame me? We'll call it my guilty pleasure.

CHAPTER TWENTY-EIGHT

NEUROTYPICAL INSINCERITY

And now for another one of my random Aspie wandering of thoughts . . .

One thing that has come to my attention over time is that some people really don't like the way we Aspies are so direct with the truth. As I mentioned in the previous chapter, Edward found me to be seriously lacking in political savvy this way. "Hold on to the information for a while. Don't say everything you're thinking." And for many others, it can be the sheer bluntness of our words that offends. I guess we do have a tendency to be brutally honest in our attempts to focus on accuracy, and sometimes we forget to consider what a person may *really* want to hear or if our words somehow constitute social taboo. People find it extremely rude and unacceptable.

However, there's a flip side to this picture. I wanted to stop for a second and talk about how neurotypicals look to us Aspies!

Have you ever noticed how often typical people say things they don't really mean? For example, when someone says, "Hi, how are you?" they don't really want to know the details of your latest dishwasher troubles and how your leg is covered in lumps from mosquito bites. They're usually just being polite.

When someone says, "Wow, what a fantastic job!" to a friend (or especially a child), it's impossible to know whether they really like the work or not. They may be saying they do regardless, because that's what typical people do with people they know!

When a friend recounts a troubling incident, have you noticed how others will gather to validate the person and tell them they were right, despite how logical or illogical their behavior really was? Those same friends could then easily talk to the other person involved and tell them they were right too. It's all about making each other feel better—support in the form of words without any real meaning. To an Aspie who values and may genuinely want to know the truth, this can all be exhausting to have to dig through!

Back before I had my first son, Isaac, I took part in an infertility forum online and found it quite eye opening to observe the "rules" of question and response. When a person posts, "Help, I am nine weeks pregnant and I just had some bleeding. It was pinkish red and has been starting and stopping lightly for two days. Is the baby going to be okay?" they don't always want to hear, "Well, there is a 50 percent chance the pregnancy will survive. Bleeding happens a lot in early pregnancy for unknown reasons. About half the time, it spontaneously stops or continues as a harmless bleed, and the other half miscarry. Only time will tell." (I've written answers like that before, and they don't seem to get responded to!)

It seems the correct answers are more along the lines of, "Great big hugs," "I feel for you honey," "Oh how awful for you to be going through this," "I'm thinking of you XOX," etc., or to recount a positive story about a friend who had bleeding and ended up with a beautiful baby! So I guess the real point of the exercise isn't fact finding but making the person feel less stressed regardless of what the truth may be, and somehow, just hearing these words does seem to work for typical people! (I have no idea how.)

To someone like me, however, this alteration in the game from fact finding to "emotional support" can be frustrating, because when I post a question, I really *do* wish to know the answer! I want the latest statistics on baby survival rates for people in my situation narrowed down by age, stage of pregnancy, hormone levels, etc., if possible. The more data, the better!

In that moment, I don't care about great big hugs or whose thoughts are with me. That doesn't help. I don't even know these respondents, so to me, it doesn't feel authentic. All I really want to know is what my odds are so I can brace myself for the outcome. Why is it so hard to get an honest answer out of people?

Similarly, if someone doesn't like me, I wish they would just tell me instead of acting like everything is fine and forcing me to work it out for myself. When I first moved to Houston, which I will talk about later, I knew a lady who, at one point, started to give me confusing signals. She would say positive, supportive words to my face with enthusiasm and a smile but in between began excluding me in a way that gave me the impression she perhaps didn't want me around. I related events over time to my friend Irene back in Australia, and we decided after a while that the lady indeed didn't seem to like me.

After one amusing conversation about it, Irene and I jokingly coined the term "snot face" to describe people who behave in this way. It wasn't because we were implying it to be something awful or the person bad. It was because if this were a childhood playground, all this confusion could've been avoided by a few simple interactions.

The lady would've poked her tongue out at me and said, "You're a snot face!" I would've replied with, "Well, you're a poo-poo head," and then it would all have been over. I would have known where I stood and could have moved on. "Snot face" became an ironic label for someone doing exactly the opposite!

I once worked out the reason I think women do this two-faced sort of behavior. It's something about keeping their place in some social hierarchy that typical people aspire to—one that I guess I fail to see or acknowledge. I suppose the more that people like you, the easier it is to maintain a good position in the eyes of others. Direct aggression could make you enemies who would find ways to bring you down. Backstabbing is a big problem. So it seems the normal way to go is to only direct your annoyance at people subtly and keep it deniable, i.e., with coolness and distance and gossip behind people's backs.

I, however, don't think in terms of hierarchy and often have trouble making sense of these ingrained behaviors. It wasn't until later in life that I even understood why people would be inconsistent in how they talk to you directly versus how they really feel.

But at least learning this has helped me understand how typical people tick and what they really want when they're upset. When I see a friend who is feeling down, I often do genuinely want to help. I do have compassion, despite what many people assume about Aspies. So if random supportive analogies and xox's is what a friend needs to feel better in a time of trouble, then so be it. Hey, it seems silly to me, but if I really can help a friend by showing support in that way, then I guess it's worth doing. Let the craziness begin!

CHAPTER TWENTY-NINE

BEING MELODRAMATIC OR OVERLY INTENSE

Q: Why do Aspies have to get so melodramatic and overly intense about things? Why can't they just make comfortable small talk like the rest of us?

I noticed recently that a particular Aspie friend of mine, David N., likes to use dramatic, highly descriptive terms when writing. He's very particular about selecting every word to make sure he gets just the right meaning and uses many words to explain himself. I quite like his expression. It's poetic and emotional. However, I guess some would find it over the top.

It reminds me of feedback I once got when writing stories for high school English. "It's good, Michelle, but a bit over emphatic. You use too many descriptive words." I recall a particular teacher once joking about me writing descriptions like "wet water" to show me how I was using words redundantly. So I wonder, why do I have that desire to pick five words of similar meaning to describe something? Why do I like to repeat my meaning in different ways? Why do I write three "why" sentences in a row?

During a discussion with this particular Aspie friend one day, I worked out that there's a likely reason behind it. I think it's that for some of us Aspies, while we feel plenty of our own emotions, it can be hard to imagine and generate the same strength of emotion just from reading or hearing the words of others.

For example, when a typical person hears a word such as "hurt," they seem to get a deeper, instant sense of grief at the other person's sorrow, whereas I don't really get that feeling until I take some time to think about it. As a writer, when I want to express "hurt," the word alone doesn't feel strong enough to convey the full impact of what I'm feeling. I'll want to say, "deeply hurt, crushed, gutted, feeling sick in the stomach and choked up," because that's what I would need to read to stir the same feelings in me. I'll want to say it again and again in different ways until the reader really knows the exact feeling. For typical people, this is redundant.

In writing this book, I've tried to be careful not to use too many words or be too repetitive in my sentiments. However, you'll have to forgive me if it's still somewhat my tendency.

For the same reason, I think that it's easy for an Aspie to sound melodramatic or overly intense when we start telling someone about our emotions or problems. While we dig straight into the heart of an issue and explain the full details of what's involved, a neurotypical might need a briefer summary with softened words to not feel overwhelmed by the emotional load.

When something is bothering me, I like to discuss the details at length. Talking things out calms me and doesn't overstimulate me in any way when either talking or listening. I find it interesting to hear others' thoughts in detail. I had no idea until recently that this could be draining or too intense for anybody. I guess that not all people can handle it the way I do!

I guess this also explains the Aspie distaste of making small talk. We find it mind numbing, lacking in content, and tiresome, because we're mainly tuning into the details and not focusing on the social or emotional purpose of the conversation, probably in the same way that typical people can find our conversation intense, overly technical, detailed, and exhausting.

For me, it's hard to come up with anything to say in a conversation that, on the whole, seems lacking in purpose. However, I've learnt that apparently, there is a purpose, and that purpose is bonding—a social dance if you will—and small talk is such a strong part of our culture that everyone is required to learn the steps of the dance and join in, typical or otherwise.

Now, to be rather quirky here, I wanted to pause and draw out the steps of this dance as I see it, because this really is how unnatural it looks to me. (Consider this my dry sense of humor.)

Example 1—The new couch dance

Step 1. Introduce random piece of information of interest to the person bringing it up. (It has to be brief.)

"Oh, guess what. We finally bought a new couch for the living room."

Step 2. Person Two provides words of enthusiasm and interest and perhaps asks a further question.

"Oh, that's great. What did you end up getting?"

Step 3. Person One provides more information on their topic of interest (making sure you don't go into any real detail).

"We picked the blue one with the lavender stripes. I was thinking it'll match the chairs in the dining room."

Step 4. More words of interest and/or further questions (no more than one or two questions at a time).

"Oh, I'm glad. I thought that one was a particularly nice choice. I think the beige might've clashed with the curtains."

Step 5. Keep repeating until sufficient enthusiasm has been shown and the topic moves on to another. Make sure to take turns as the topic-raiser.

"I was thinking that myself . . . etc."

And rather importantly, you must always stick to the rules of the dance; i.e., never go too far in one direction, for fear of hitting a wall. Turn around and change topic frequently. Keep it light. Keep it happy. Definitely avoid elaborating on any negative thoughts or feelings. Always smile, look at your dance partner, and remain engaged!

To mess with your mind even further, in girl-world, I've also come across an alternative version of the dance with a more sophisticated beginning:

Example 2—The new couch dance: The ladies' version

Step 1. You guess what the other person might want to talk about based on what you know about them or sense they might be feeling.

"So, did you have any luck looking for couches?"

Step 2. They provide a one- or two-sentence answer to the topic at hand.

"Oh, we finally bought a new one for the living room. I was so happy to see it arrive. It took three weeks for delivery even though the shop is only over in Spainsburry Street. I had to ring them twice to find out when it was coming."

Step 3. Move to step two of the original dance and continue.

This extra step, I'm led to understand, is a way to communicate sufficient *interest* in your friends and their lives. Not only should you be thinking about them, but you're expected to show you are thinking about them and their lives by playing "Guess what topics they might want to talk about." And all this time, here I was just trying to do my simple Aspie dance instead:

Example 3—My Aspie dance

Step 1. I talk about my topics, and you listen and reply.

"Hooray. I just finished revising Chapter Forty-Nine of my book. Forty-nine down, seven left to go. You know, one day I may actually get through this thing!"

Step 2. You talk about your topics, and I listen and reply.

"By the way, yesterday I went shopping and found that new couch I'd been looking for."

No wonder so many women don't find my mode of conversation satisfactory!

If you can't tell, I'm saying the above a bit tongue-in-cheek. To me, adding this extra questioning requirement is just making it all too complicated, and I don't have the energy to always be doing that. I'll question at times when my friends' lives are on my mind, and at other times I probably won't. So please don't take my lack of asking about things personally. It's just something I'll need to practice more to get in the habit of doing.

But I do raise this topic seriously, as it can genuinely cause problems when some women want to talk about themselves but wait for lead-ins to do so. There are women out there who don't like to raise their own topics too much, as they fear it would be impolite, and find our failure to question annoying. So all I can do is apologize for that. I am trying!

(And a hint from an Aspie to typical people who feel that way: there's something you can do about this situation. If you want to talk about yourself to an Aspie and feel uncomfortable raising a topic, just do it anyway! We don't care how often you bring your issues up. And quite frankly, waiting for a polite invitation from us might take all year!)

Anyway, going back to the typical-people bonding dance, I did want to address a few missteps that I've noticed Aspies commonly make, because I think having a basic understanding of these could aid NT-Aspie communication a lot. So, for the Aspies out there, here is my top mistakes list:

> **Misstep 1:** Responding to the topic by relating an experience of our own (too frequently).

As an Aspie, it feels natural to respond to a conversation by relating our experiences, especially when the topic is emotional. We're basically saying, "I know how you feel/what you are experiencing because I've had a feeling/experience like that myself." To us, it's a display that we're actually connecting to a person's feelings and are bonding with them.

However, typical people don't need to have had a similar experience to feel what a friend might be feeling, and they don't need to relate that experience to show they understand. Changing the topic this way on occasion is fine, but when we do it frequently, all a typical person hears is, "me me me." They assume our genuine attempts to connect are displays of selfishness, and it puts them off talking to us. Unfortunately, this is a common misunderstanding.

> **Misstep 2:** Going into too much detail.

This one is self-explanatory. Typical people don't want to hear too much technical detail when focusing on their social dance. It makes them think and tires them out, when they aren't really up for "working." They are busy focusing on bonding and putting all their energy into social connection. (Regardless of the fact that this bonding exercise is completely mind-numbing for us, leaving us craving more intellectual conversation).

> **Misstep 3:** Focusing on the details of the topic instead of the emotional words

When a typical person throws in a subtle emotional word, they expect us to empathize and feel that word and respond to it regardless of what other information they've conveyed. If we miss the emotional words and respond about the other details instead, they feel invalidated, and it's easy for Aspies to miss these things when typical people throw them out so subtly.

For example, when someone says, "Oh, I'm so stressed. The car lock had frosted inside, so I had to wait to start the car," "stressed" is the key word, so don't make your only response, "Did you try using water?"

And so, that concludes our discussion today on the dance of the neurotypicals, leaving us poor Aspies wishing we could just get out of there and run far, far away!! It's one of the many downsides of being a minority in a neurotypical world. We have to learn the local culture. The onus is on us.

And I've definitely had times where I've amused myself by imagining a world that was the other way around, where Aspies defined the cultural norms, where we could skip all formalities or discussions of topics that disinterested us. We could walk into shops without being bothered by sales people and focus on the process of actually buying what we were trying to buy, with the shelves all lined out sequentially in a logical order by product type and details. We could approach friends directly with questions on what we wanted to know; i.e., no, "Hi, how are you?" Just walk up and say, "What color ink cartridges does your printer use?"

At functions, we'd be left in peace to eat the food and listen to the music and only talk when we were inclined to. When we did talk, the discussions would be so heavy and interesting that we would actually want to engage. The atmosphere would be restful. The light would be dimmed. I know that to me, an Aspie-majority world sounds enticing. I wonder if other Aspies find this idea similarly appealing.

CHAPTER THIRTY

LIFE AFTER FULL-TIME WORK: MY EXPERIENCE IN CHILDCARE

Okay, so after having quit Valcorp, I decided that I really didn't want to go back into the engineering world or any type of full-time work again—for real this time! My problems in the workplace were something that I still didn't fully understand, but it was clear that whatever was going on, being in a nine-to-five job had a way of leaving me void. And the more time I had to pause and really feel what I'd gone through, the more I could see just how shut down and damaged I'd become from such prolonged stress. I'd come out of the workplace like a train wreck, and I didn't want to put myself in any environment that could do that to me again.

Being the driven person that I am, I became focused immediately on what I *should* do next. Naturally, I had to have a job. More than that, I needed a long-term plan and goals. But nothing I could think of felt like it was going to be better. Perhaps I needed something simpler, I thought to myself. Perhaps I just needed to do a more mundane job. So I spent a little time looking for part time-work that I thought might be okay as a simple job on the side.

However, after sending in applications for a dozen or so part-time roles and having several interviews, the answer always seemed to be the same: I was overqualified. I guess the employers didn't see me as a serious candidate who was going to stay in the role, and in hindsight, I guess they were probably right. I wasn't really ready to re-enter the workforce yet. Who knows how long I would have stayed? It left me in limbo, unsure of my next move. Oh, how I hated being in that limbo.

In the back of my mind, I also spent a lot of time thinking about how much I wanted to start a family and began to try to do so during this time. But things didn't seem to be happening for me quickly, and it became clear after a while that those plans were going to have to wait. Could I not fall pregnant at all? No, I refused to accept that, and later on after the mandatory year of trying, I turned to a fertility specialist to begin the process of testing for issues and taking fertility medication. Everything came up clear, and it was puzzling why things were just not happening for me.

I saw a lady who counseled me briefly over that time, which helped me a lot to find a little of myself again. In particular, I remember one thing she said to me that really changed my perspective on seeking work. She pointed out that I wanted to work because I was running away from something—away from social pressures and being depicted as lazy or a non-contributor in society, not allowing anyone to think poorly of me. But that's not a good motivation to start anything. The right motivation to do something is from a place of stability toward something I *want* to do.

She also pointed out to me that I didn't *have* to work. I was married, and we had enough income to get by. Puzzled, I replied that I thought it was unacceptable for me to just depend on someone and not give back. How could I accept myself that way? To even consider it for a while, I needed someone to tell me that would be okay. She asked, if she gave me her permission not to work, would that make it okay, and I realized no. She asked how many people would need to give me permission not to work for it to be okay, and I said, "All of them."

And then I realized the true answer to be only one—myself. I decided to just sit with the idea for a while, and instead of aggressively searching for a job, work on finding myself again, to let the goals and dreams come to me.

Shortly after making that decision, I came up with the idea that I might like to study childcare while waiting to start my own family. I wasn't sure I had ever seen examples of great parenting, and I wanted to know how to do it better for my children, so I enrolled myself in a six-month course with childcare placements two days a week and began a Certificate III in Children's Services.

I guess in the back of my mind, I also still had the notion that this could be a way to get part-time work. Even though I was trying to let go of the work idea, I would've felt too guilty to justify the cost otherwise. So you can give me a slap on the wrist for that! I couldn't help myself. It gave me something to look forward to and that feeling I love of going somewhere with my life again.

Thrown back into the study environment, I thrived once more. My work was of high quality, and the teacher praised me for thinking outside the box and giving mature, well-considered answers to problems. Socially, I found myself a central member of the small group of women who made up the class and felt popular and admired by others. The group was culturally diverse, and I think that may have helped me fit in so well. I've read before that sometimes Aspies can fit in well in other cultures because any nuances in behavior may be dismissed as cultural differences.

The teacher was fantastic and made the class fun with more interactive lessons and a chance for a little play and silliness. For this six months of my life, I was really, really happy again.

And then, in what felt like so little time, the course was over, and I found myself back in employment limbo. Just like that. I remember how, in my exit interview with the teacher, I'd emphasized to her how I was going to miss the group and coming in to study each day. It wasn't just a thankful comment. It was almost pleading. In reply, she said in a bubbly way, "But look on the bright side. Now you get to work!" And there was that sinking gut feeling again.

Instinctively, I knew that work would only make me unhappy. She and my other classmates thought it was an exciting thing to look forward to. I couldn't explain why I didn't feel the same way. And then after the interview, it was just me again. No more fun classes again or people to see each day. I was back to where I had started.

Pregnancy-wise, I'd still failed to conceive for the duration of the course, even on fertility medication, and was starting to lose hope about it ever happening. The concept of potentially growing up childless, when I'd always seen myself as a family person, was devastating and gradually left me more and more depressed with each negative test. Infertility has a way of making you question your whole existence. What's the point if I can't have children? Isn't it the whole biological purpose of life?

This is a topic that I could write a whole book on alone, as those who have suffered from infertility know. It can become the center of all your focus and a real sore point over time. But I'll spare you that degree of melancholy.

My next attempt to get out of limbo was to follow along with what my classmates were all doing and give working in childcare a try. After all, it was a simple job—the type I'd been after before—and had part-time options. So I applied for a role with a temporary agency that served many high-quality childcare centers in my area. My classmates had tipped me off that this one, McArthur, was a particularly nice place to work if you could get in. The agency was prestigious and required a full interview plus at least a Certificate III and good references.

Fortunately, my placement references were excellent, and I was accepted quickly. The staff at the agency treated me well, allowing me to pick and choose the days that I pleased. I really couldn't say anything bad about them.

At first, I opted to work just three to four days a week, usually only half days. It was great that I was able to pick my hours each week. The agency would call me up each week with the addresses and shift times, and in I would go. It was as easy as being able to drive to a new location and then just sit and help out with the kids as directed. But very quickly, something was not right again. Ugh. Those old feelings of workplace dread started to re-emerge, much to my dismay.

I thought, "How could this be? This is an easy job and requires little mental effort. That was supposed to make the difference." But the feelings were unmistakable—exhaustion, anxiety, and feeling sick in the gut both at the idea of going in and while I was there.

I remember one particular day that I found the most unpleasant of all. The center I was at was holding a puppet show for the parents and children in celebration of a special event. The crowd gathered in the one room to watch this display, which was extremely creative, with spectacular lighting and images. It would've been enjoyable. All I had to do was sit there and make up staff numbers, really, but all I could think about was how I wanted to run out of the room—the noise, the crowd, my growing self-consciousness.

Trying to analyze what the parents, who had paid for me to be there, would think of me sitting and doing nothing, I was struggling to figure out what I should appear to be doing. Where to look. To make eye contact with people or not. How to remain alert and concentrate on what the children in the room were doing (after all, that is what I was being paid for) while watching the show at the same time. I couldn't do both, so I opted to tune out of the show and focus on "behaving right." I was so glad when the day was over. I went home feeling quite unwell. I think this was the time in my life when the social anxiety had become the worst.

It was all so frustrating. The kids were lovely, and I loved being left in the childcare room when it was just me and a few little ones. Heck, I even liked getting laundry duty when I was left alone. I loved folding such cute baby clothes and sheets. I wanted a job just doing laundry. I wished I could just be okay there in general. Why couldn't I feel okay?

Most of the centers that I went to were lovely places and probably have been great to work at had I found a way to settle there in a room that didn't stress me. But I also encountered one or two that disturbed me. I recall an experience with one child in particular. Upon entering the room, I was introduced to him with, "This is Miles. You'll get to know him. He's trouble." He looked up at me as an innocent two-year-old—big blue eyes, curly blonde hair, curious, no malice.

Mid-morning during play time in the room, there was a minor incident with Miles pulling out some blocks that he wasn't supposed to touch. The carer snapped at him to put them away, but he refused and threw a few of them instead. He was told to sit in the block corner indefinitely until he had packed them all away, but of course, this was a two-year-old. Of course he wouldn't, so a standoff was created.

The carer downright refused to let him out, and he refused to pick up any of the blocks. It went on so long that it caused him to miss his morning tea.[34] Then the carer even took a toy of his from home and pretended to throw it in the bin. It didn't motivate him at all.

Later in the day, another substitute carer and I had difficulty getting Miles to sit at the lunch table. The main carer was on a break, so I was free to interact with the children my own way and went about trying to calm him. I picked up a fish toy and said to him, "If you sit at the table nicely, I'll let you play with this fish. Do you want the fish?" He said yes. Surprisingly, he cooperated. He sat nicely while he ate his lunch, dipping the fish in and out of the empty part of his water glass.

When the main carer returned to the room, however, she shook her head and snatched the fish off him with a few words of disapproval. Miles screamed. I tried to protest that I'd given the fish to him, but she said, "It doesn't matter. He needs to learn to sit at the table without toys like the rest of the children. Don't worry about giving it to him. He'll forget in two minutes."

Why does he need to learn so fast, I thought to myself. Why can't we start where he is and move in baby steps in the right direction? But I didn't argue. It wouldn't have achieved anything. Miles protested so much that he was put in the corner. The other children in the room were told, "Miles is misbehaving again."

The next day when I came back, I gave Miles quite a bit of attention in the form of fun and play. He was skeptical at first, but he came around, and by the afternoon, he was packing up balls for me. I pointed it out to the main carer, thinking what a positive thing it was. Miles was cleaning up! But she replied with something accusing along the lines of, "Ah, so he *can* pack up. Interesting that he will do it for *you*."

What I find interesting is that when I tried to show her, "Look, you treat him the right way, and he responds," she interpreted it as, "He really is a ratbag. His defiance is on purpose." I didn't try and explain the concept any further. She wasn't going to get it.

I still think about Miles sometimes. It haunts me. How did he grow up? Did he learn to go through life fighting with everyone? Did he learn the assumption that life sucks and that people are going to treat you like crap, so you just have to take what you can get? After all, I learnt in my course that most of our major life assumptions (such as that one) are made when we're around two years old. That young! Back then, he had so much potential for it to be all turned around. I wonder now if his life is scarred because of selfish intolerance from his carers that he received before it was even in his control.

In the same center (another room) one morning, I found a baby sitting on the floor crying, a little Indian boy or girl (I couldn't really tell). I went to pick the child up and

---

[34] Morning tea = morning snack

was told not to bother. "That child cries all day unless it's carried. It needs to learn to play on its own." I couldn't stomach leaving the child. I was defiant (a rare moment for me) and picked the child up anyway until it was comforted. I guess I didn't help it in the long run.

And so it continued. I could write a few more stories about the same sort of thing (and I actually did in the first draft!), but I think you get the point. So I'll move on!

After finishing my Certificate III, I ended up working in this temp role for around five or six months and went to perhaps twenty or thirty centers. Some I imagine I could've been happy in had I been able to settle in okay in a part-time, comfortable role. However, at least as a temp, those stress feelings really started to gnaw at me, so I slowly cut down my days per week until eventually I decided the stress was just too unpleasant to cope with and suspended coming in entirely. I told the agency I was "unavailable indefinitely" and never did end up going back. I knew something was just wrong with me in the workplace. I needed to figure out what.

As an excuse—probably more to myself than others—I told people I was going to stop work for a while to focus on fertility treatment, as all the stress probably wasn't helping with that. I went in to have laparoscopic surgery, and the doctor removed some endometriosis. Then I went back on fertility meds that I was only supposed to take for up to four months because, apparently, if it doesn't happen by then, it's not going to, and the meds are unhealthy long term.

After the third month, still nothing, and I gave up and prepared myself mentally for starting full-blown IVF. Given my particular issues, there was no guarantee it would work any better than the meds, but I was running out of other choices. And then on the fourth month, out of the blue, the most wonderful thing happened. After eighteen months of trying and undergoing fertility treatment, I was finally fortunate enough to conceive my first son, Isaac.

The news was amazing and quite unbelievable to me. Being off work at the time, I was relaxed and free to have a most enjoyable pregnancy, and I went about reveling in my new obsession of reading up on baby books and parenting advice. You can imagine how fixated on it I became! Two years later, with a few more fertility meds, I was then blessed with another baby boy, Trent, and have remained a stay-at-home mum ever since.

And what can I say but that after having my boys, all those silly worries about being in limbo and what other people think just melted away and became unimportant. Who cares what society thinks of me when I have my boys to think about? They're the most precious things in my life and the only ones that really matter in the long run. And I'm so glad I was *finally* able to mature in that way!

But don't assume my story is over just yet. It turns out that parenting and dealing with other mothers was a brand new ballpark for me, and I had a lot more uncomfortable social lessons to learn.

To be continued . . .

Chapter Thirty-One

Female versus Male Diagnosis

Q: So I've heard that the ratio of Autism in men and women is something like four to one. Why do you think there are so many more men diagnosed than women?

Ah, yes. The staggering difference between the number of girls diagnosed with Autism and Asperger's and the number of boys is something that has been puzzling scientists for years.

It makes you question, are there really more men with Asperger's than women, or are the women simply falling under the radar? And I have to confess, I don't know the scientific answer to this, as studies on the topic are still rather inconclusive. However, my personal suspicions are that it's more to do with the latter. Women with Asperger's just don't seem to stand out as much as our male counterparts, because our style of oddness is more commonplace and easier to miss.

I read an article just recently in which a mother of two children on the spectrum, Annette Lewns, explained that while her Autistic son was picked up at age three, her similarly afflicted daughter was unable to get the help she needed until she was nine years of age! She writes, "The doctors failed time and time again to see through her coping strategies. I fought for years, but I was confronted with a wall of disbelief and skepticism. They were simply unable to understand that a girl might present differently to a boy."[35]

As a condition that was historically described as "extreme maleness,"[36] Autism in a boy can make an individual seem extreme, an outlier on the charts of what's considered "normal" behavior, whereas women can be more of a mixed bag of "unusual." We may come across as odd, more rational/logical in our thinking, less empathetic, quirky, and/or "not really like the other girls," but we don't fall so far out of the realm of "normal" human behavior as to be flagged. We are still, in part, female and show some degree of social coherence.

Compounding this problem further is the fact that diagnosed Aspie women are relatively rare and thorough studies on Autism in women are lacking. Historically, Asperger's was always seen as a male condition, and in the days of early Asperger's research, women were often removed from studies altogether as we tended to "muddy up the data."[37] This means that much of our current understanding on Autistic behavior is based on studies of males only, and our diagnostic tools are tailored specifically to diagnose men, so it's no wonder that the females are being overlooked!

And whether it's a good thing or to our own detriment, I think women are just inclined to care more about what other people think, so we may put more work into the act of blending in and compensating for our differences. The result of these factors combined is someone whose behavior doesn't jump out as strongly abnormal to the casual observer.

So does this mean that women's Asperger's is milder or that women don't need as much help as the men do? No, I wouldn't say so. Women with Asperger's, or high-functioning individuals in general, often still suffer from the same difficulties that someone of lower functioning may—difficulties in perceiving social cues or reading body language, frustration from oversensitivity or interruptions of hyperfocus, etc.

It just means that instead of expressing these difficulties as outward behavior, we work harder to suppress them and are suffering in more internal ways instead. It's similar to the difference between anger and depression. One causes the people around us to suffer, and the other causes us to struggle in silence.

---

[35] Landon Bryce, "How We Fail Girls and Women," The Autcast, 17 April 2012, http://thautcast.com/drupal5/content/how-we-fail-autistic-girls-and-women

[36] Baron-Cohen, S., "The extreme male brain theory of Autism," In: Tager-Flusberg, Helen, (Editor) "Neurodevelopmental Disorders," MIT Press, Cambridge, MA, 1999, pp. 401-429

[37] Janeen Interlandi, "More Than Just 'Quirky'," The Daily Beast, Nov 12, 2008 7:00 PM EST http://www.thedailybeast.com/newsweek/2008/11/12/more-than-just-quirky.html

I think it's true that people on the highest functioning end of the spectrum can have the hardest time with their Autism, because people around us don't recognize the cause of our difficulties and are more likely to misunderstand and mistreat us. We don't wear a sign on our heads saying, "I have Asperger's Syndrome (or HFA). Please take that into consideration before you go making assumptions about me." When we try to fit in, people don't always see the whole picture. They don't realize how much work we are already putting in just to pass as we are.

I think it's important to keep in mind that when we define the severity of a person's Autism, it's *only* a measure of outward behavior and doesn't really reflect how much one is affected by the condition internally. Those of us who appear to have low severity may actually need more than is apparent to the eye. So it would be good if there were more emotional outreach and assessment for these people, because, as it is, I think the silent sufferers still remain strongly undersupported.

CHAPTER THIRTY-TWO

STIMMING

Q: Someone mentioned to me that a lot of people on the Autism spectrum stim. What is stimming, and what are your stims?

Stimming is the action of making repetitive motions such as flapping or rocking to self-sooth and mentally stimulate the brain. And yes, it is extremely common in Autistics and presents in some Aspies too.

For me, stimming isn't something that I ever thought about much, because I haven't experienced it noticeably. I always imagined stims as big, obvious, odd-looking movements for those with little self-awareness, which didn't sound like me at all. However, I've learnt during my Aspie journey that not all forms of stimming are obvious.

For example, stims can be subtle things such as pacing or circling one's fingers repeatedly, and some people are never consciously aware they're doing them. Yes, even relatively normal people—well, as normal as me anyway! Then there are others who are aware of their stims but have learnt to hide them or disguise them as something else, such as coughing or moving to music. I have a friend who likes to push his glasses up his nose to hide the fact that he has a nose-rubbing type of stim. It takes away the impression of anything being "odd." So stims are definitely not just something for the severely impaired like I once imagined.

Learning more, it turns out that a few little things I do, like bouncing my leg under the table or singing repeatedly to myself do actually have a stimming purpose. It's interesting that I never identified these behaviors as stimming before, because I was aware they were odd and not for public viewing. I've always made a point to keep them subtle or not to do them in public, and I've been doing that as long as I can remember. I guess I just put it down to private habits.

But now that I know that stimming exists, I can see that it can appear in a range of ways, both major and minor. So, for your information, here are some of the most common types of stims:

- Flapping
- Rocking
- Bouncing
- Spinning
- Jumping
- Pacing
- Toe walking
- Lining up objects
- Singing or humming
- Grunting
- Making vocal sounds repeatedly
- Clapping
- Opening and closing fists
- Snapping fingers
- Twiddling fingers
- Tapping fingers
- Nail biting
- Hair twisting
- Scratching
- Feeling objects
- Rubbing skin
- Sniffing
- Chewing the inside of lips or mouth
- Grinding teeth
- Running tongue around an object in your mouth
- Sucking on things
- Staring at lights
- Blinking
- Gazing at fingers

And I have to say, some of those surprised me. Who knew that twirling my hair could be a stim? In fact, that could explain a lot!

I had an interesting experience pointing out a stim to an Aspie friend of mine, John, not too long ago. When sitting with him at a dinner out, I noticed that he tended to bounce up and down slightly in his seat when bored or restless. I suggested to him that it looked like it could be a type of stim.

It's such a simple thing, but he was fascinated by the realization. I assume he'd never before been consciously aware that he did bounce and/or that other people didn't in the same manner. I wonder how many other Aspies have little stims they don't even know about.

CHAPTER THIRTY-THREE

LIFE IN MELBOURNE, PRE-HOUSTON

Q: So, after you walked away from childcare, what did you do with yourself next?

Oh, you have no idea how wonderful it felt that day that I walked away from my workplace again, this time *actually* for the last time.

No more work now. I just wanted to be free to be me—free to think about what I wanted to when I wanted to without my brain being exhausted and tied up on other tasks and free to have some space to allow my Aspie inspiration to bloom.

Of course, at first it wasn't exactly the smoothest transition for me to go from being busy to having all the time in the world. I wasn't completely sure what to do with myself, and I wandered around sort of lost for some months—even a year—after I ceased work. Transitions can be tough, but at least the break afforded me a lot of spare time to ponder, and I took to spending periods of time just sitting and reflecting outside with the trees and greenery like I used to do in my pre-work days.

It was almost a meditative activity that I'd dearly missed, and it helped to soothe and calm me. I felt at home out with nature, laying on my back, watching the clouds go by and the movement of the leaves above, just thinking.

I do recall, one thing that I thought about a lot in this time was how the world "ought" to work and where I fit in. For the first time—ever, really—I'd lost my attachment to that nine-to-five "study, work, succeed" pathway that I'd always believed to be the right way to do things, and I found myself questioning what I really wanted. What were the things that were truly important to me in life, and what did I want to become?

I started to see that life isn't about what you do. It's about who you are and what you love, and the true goal should simply be to make yourself and others happy, perhaps balancing the present and the future, but not with so much focus on money, recognition, status, or power. People get so caught up in the pursuit of these things that they fail to value the truly meaningful things in life. I think it's unfortunate that this society puts so much focus on a person's working role and money-earning potential as the basis of their identity. It fails to value all the other things that a person has to contribute.

I'm glad that I eventually reached a point where I began to open my mind and question the idea of what success is and what is really important in life and happiness. It's just a shame that, for me, this process had to stem from failure.

Anyway, not to bore you . . .

I began to make a point of seeking out all the little things in life that brought me joy. I looked up clubs, activity groups, and Meetup.com sites. I Googled what volunteer work was available in the area, any ideas to get me up and going with . . . something. But it was difficult, because I'd shut off a lot of the things I loved while working when they didn't seem important at the time. I struggled to find anything that made me feel enthusiastic. I didn't know who I was any more.

One thing that became clear rather quickly, however, was that I was a social being, and connection with others was critical to my happiness, so I began to look purposefully for ways to establish new and rewarding friendships.

I joined a "girls' group" that met up every Thursday evening, which was a rather unconventional thing for me to do. The group was religion-based and alternated between social activities and worship, and I wasn't really a believer. But the girls were nice to me, and I valued the social interaction, so I was happy to take what I could get. There was no requirement for me to pretend to be religious or anything but myself, and the group counseled one another and gave each other support in a way that I think is invaluable.

I've heard people indicate before that seeing a professional is the ticket to solve any issue, but sometimes I think that a good set of friends and a support network is just as vital, if not more, and no professional counselor can ever replace the absence of that.

I'd first heard about Girls' Group when my friend Emma from high school ran a course on boundaries in relationships. She'd become a psychologist later in life and knew I took interest in general psychological issues. She thought that I might enjoy the subject matter and invited me along to study with the girls. During those twelve weeks or so, I had some enjoyable, in-depth conversations with the girls during the discussion groups. We opened up a lot about some personal issues, and I made some strong con-nections.

After the course ended, I remember commenting how much I'd enjoyed seeing everyone weekly and was going to miss the group. So they invited me to keep coming to their Girls' Group, the more religious-based gathering. It was probably the first time in my life that I'd ever made solid female friends.

I also began to see one lady, Jo, regularly outside the group, visiting her house with Isaac on the odd weekday. She had a young daughter of her own and was just overcom-ing a long battle with post-natal depression, making us good companions to lean on each other. We set up regular play dates, which made it into a comfortable, routine activity for me. Though we differed greatly in social ability, Jo was kind, loyal, protec-tive, motherly, and a supportive neurotypical friend.

I've read articles before on how Aspie girls cope in high school, and I understand that one common theme is girls finding themselves under the wing of a protective, mothering type who shields them from social difficulty. I'd never had anyone in high school play that role for me, but if anyone I know would fit that personality type, it would be Jo.

In one particular Girls' Group memory that stands out in my mind, I commented to the group that I needed to find more friends and asked how I should go about seek-ing them out. I thought I needed additional friends for when these friends ran out—backup friends or friends to rotate between. I raised this to the group as a topic.

In this discussion, I remember one lady asking me, "Why do you need additional friends? You'll always have us." And I think that moment was the first time in my life I felt like I might be in a stable friend situation. The comment really resonated with me and played over in my mind. These girls wanted to be part of my life indefinitely. Maybe I didn't have to be so insecure any longer.

In the past, I guess I had a few too many experiences where people seemed to get sick of me and fade out over time. The notion that someone who knew me well could be talking to me about remaining friends forever was very novel indeed.

In the Girls' Group, it was okay, it seemed, to be a little bit myself. The girls were patient and non-judgmental, and I could tell them things. It was a really affirm-ing experience. Perhaps, secretly, some of the girls may have been holding onto hope that I would eventually turn religious too by partaking in the group. However, I think they'd have stayed my friends regardless.

When I announced that I was pregnant, the girls were thrilled for me, and two of the ladies, Jo and Sarah, threw me a fantastic baby shower. They made me feel loved and confident that the baby would be wanted, and I, in Aspie style, became obsessed with discussing my new Vines-to-be.

At the same point in time, Robert and I also reconnected with a group of two couples that he knew from high school. Robert invited the guys over for a boys' night when I went to Girls' Group to watch movies and eat nachos, and through the odd group event, we all got to know each other better with time. As couples, we started going on the occasional holiday together, which was always fantastic.

These people felt more "like" to me than anyone else in my life ever had, and I was able to enjoy the conversation as a part of the group rather than someone sitting on the outside listening in. I looked forward to our gatherings. I suspect that perhaps I wasn't the only Aspie in the mix.

In addition to these critical friends, I'd also formed a relationship with my sister-in-law, who had her own baby son. I also had a supportive set of parents on both sides (Isaac's grandparents) and a brother-in-law on my husband's side with a wife and two young children of his own. Heck, I'd even formed friends in the new mothers' group at the local child health center. I had the good fortune to be placed with some particularly kind and friendly ladies for parenting sessions after Isaac was born.

To a typical person reading this, I suppose you might wonder why I would tell you about all these people. Usually, such a network of friendships is easy to obtain, and discussing it may seem mundane. But to me, as an Aspie, finding that small number of people with whom I can connect has always been like finding the few needles in a large haystack. Arriving at this point was quite a journey.

Unfortunately, this time in Ormond (Melbourne) was short lived, and after only a year and a half of being free from the workforce, my husband and I moved to Houston, Texas. But I mention this time in my life because I think it was so important to me in terms of self-esteem and emotional stability. Having positive, supportive neurotypical friends back in Australia taught me a fundamental lesson: that I am acceptable and valuable as I am and don't need to change for anybody but myself.

Without having had this experience, I honestly don't know how I would've gotten through the harder times ahead. Sometimes, just having someone online saying, "No, Michelle, so-and-so is being mean. There's nothing wrong with you as you are, and you don't have to change to please them," was invaluable. I would like to particularly thank my friend Irene (out of the two couples) for getting me through a very rough patch. Friendships like these are like gold and should always be treasured. I think every Aspie needs at least one or two of these types of people in their life. If only they were easy to find!

And it was these sorts of friendships that I was definitely going to need to cope with my life in Houston and the harder times that I was about to face! But again, more about that later . . .

CHAPTER THIRTY-FOUR

ASPERGER'S SYNDROME AND BEING LONELY

I think it's a common misconception that because someone has Autism or Asperger's Syndrome, they're fine with (or even prefer) being alone for long periods. It's true that we Aspies do have a higher tolerance for being by ourselves than most and can very much enjoy having downtime to focus on our own things, but for me, there's definitely a limit to how much isolation I can stand, and I know I'm not the only Aspie who feels this social need.

Despite our tendency to appear aloof or disinterested, we Aspies are still social creatures with real human needs. We need company and companionship as much as anyone else does, at least in the right quantities given our lifestyle.

Now, I know that for some Aspies, that quantity appears to be zero, zilch, zip! Yep, there's always an Aspie I bump into here or there who talks about how they've just had enough of people and wish that everyone would just leave them alone and stop pressuring them to go to things. (It's usually said in a grumpy tone!) But you have to consider how much time a person already spends around others in their day-to-day lives; i.e., work, home life, hobbies, etc.

I, too, remember how, back in the days when I was studying and working, I had no real desire for social contact at all. The day-after-day exhaustion of dealing with strangers and colleagues more than filled my desire for socialization, and in my downtime, I just needed to recharge. An occasional lunch with my friends was enjoyable, but a party after work? Forget it, unless you were someone I was really close to and the group was small.

Sometimes I would go to these things because I felt an obligation to for one reason or another, but rarely for pleasure. Heck, when I was working in the city, sometimes I would even go find a quiet staircase in the train station at lunch just to be where nobody else was. Back then, I really appreciated the time I had to just sit with my own thoughts or work on little things that were important to me.

Then I ceased working, and I was thrown into a whole different world.

Admittedly, for the first few weeks, it was bliss—endless hours of precious alone time for me. But soon after, the boredom and isolation set in. I needed stimulation. I needed someone to talk to, to air all these thoughts in my head. Being alone for days on end is like torture.

I'm not just being melodramatic. It can really make you start to go crazy, and I don't think people can fully understand the strength of this frustration until they've experienced it for themselves. It leads rapidly to depression, not unlike solitary confinement. I never thought that I was the kind of person who would feel that way, but it turns out I am.

Later, wandering on to the online Aspie forums, I was surprised to discover that it wasn't just me who felt that way. There are so many desperately lonely Aspies out there, writing post after post of bleak and intense stories in which other people are rejecting them—posts about those who they thought were friends walking away, posts about those new people they wanted to get to know but never found a way to approach.

I read a handful of suicidal posts from those who were so painfully alone, they didn't want to go on. And all I could do was empathize. Yes, an Aspie empathizing. Because these were feelings I could relate to and therefore understand.

I remember writing, myself, once about how sometimes I feel as if I'm in a glass box. I know the world is out there. I can see it, in a blurry way, through the glass. I can hear muffled sounds and the laughter of others, and I know there are things I would want to be a part of—special interest groups, social organizations, gatherings that are right for me—but I have no idea how to find them or reach them, as I'm trapped in this cage.

How do people know where to go and what to do? What events are coming up? I browsed the internet endlessly but came up with little that is realistic. I guess most small, private events that I would enjoy aren't advertised there. Is it word of mouth? I'm generally out of that loop. Another lady wrote about how she felt trapped in a glass jar and couldn't get the lid off or keep it off. It was a similar analogy to mine.

I remember writing in another post about how I sometimes felt I had a voice in my head just screaming and how I couldn't go to sleep because the screaming was too loud. Of course, it wasn't a real voice (I don't hallucinate). It was more an auditory representation that perfectly described a feeling or frustration I felt and couldn't otherwise express. The feeling was so strong, I couldn't tune it out.

Upon writing this, I'm happy to relay that I haven't had this feeling in a long time. My life has picked up a lot since that point, and I have a few close people I can reach out to now. It's not the problem that it used to be, but sometimes I think of how many others must still be suffering out there, isolated and alone. Too many. I wish there was something we could do to fix this.

CHAPTER THIRTY-FIVE

WHAT IS ASPERGER'S SYNDROME?

Q: You keep talking about what it's like to have Asperger's Syndrome and you call yourself an Aspie. But what is Asperger's Syndrome?

Well, that's a good question. As I addressed in the foreword, I left this question until quite late in the book, because I wanted to give you a chance to first see me as a person—a complete person who isn't just somebody with a "syndrome."

And I wanted to avoid people simply dismissing me as "different" before even giving me a chance. Not that you weren't aware I had Asperger's, of course, but at least I avoided defining myself with a list of symptoms that you would look for as you read the book.

But I think I've spent enough time chatting to you now that I'm ready to give my thoughts on the topic (even though you haven't been awfully talkative back!). So, then, what is Asperger's Syndrome?

Well, to my understanding, Asperger's is basically a condition where the brain grows and develops in different ways than that of a typical person. It becomes overdeveloped in some areas and underdeveloped in others, not unlike the way in which the male and female brain grow differently.

For example—to get all scientific on you for a minute—when the female brain grows, it develops a larger network of interconnecting tissue within the brain (more white matter)[38] and a larger connecting structure (the corpus callosum).[39] This means women can transfer data between the two sides of the brain faster than men[40] and can use both sides of the brain more evenly. These additional interconnections make women naturally better at things like multitasking, subtleties in communication, verbal abilities, empathizing, and other typical female traits.

The male brain, on the other hand, grows less interconnecting tissue and focuses its growth on more densely developed processing tissue (more grey matter)."[41]" Males approach tasks with a single hemisphere of the brain predominating. These differences make males naturally better at things like logic, systemizing, problem solving, spatial awareness, and mental rotation of objects.

In a similar manner, the Asperger's brain grows in a way that makes us particularly strong in logical and technical thinking, rationality, intense focus, and perhaps mathematics, sciences, music, and/or arts, depending on the individual.

The downside is that we're less in tune in areas of social functions such as reading between the lines, understanding body language, knowing when to speak or what's appropriate to say, following fashions, and social cues in general. Studies on brain growth in Asperger's are still a new thing, and the cause for these differences are only beginning to be understood, but already, some noticeable differences have been picked up.

Anyway, to avoid boring you too much, I won't rattle off any further technical details here, but for those who are interested, I've included a summary table in the appendix of the brain differences found so far as I understand them (Appendix One).

And note—disclaimer! disclaimer!—I made this table back in 2012, so it is probably out of date, and I'm no expert on brain structure. It mixes Asperger's and Autism studies and doesn't detail what was done in each study. So if you want more accurate, up-to-date information—and are someone who can actually be bothered reading scientific documents!—please follow the links and investigate for yourself! I designed this as just a summary table to help people pick up Autistic neurology at a glance.

And I don't know if you take as much interest in these technicalities as I do, but my thoughts on the table are, "Wow, isn't it fascinating? The subjects with Autism

---

[38,41] Haier, Richard et. al., "The neuroanatomy of general intelligence: sex matters," NeuroImage, Volume 25, Issue 1, Pages 320–327, March 2005, quoted in: Carey, Bjorn. 'Men and Women Really Do Think Differently.' LiveScience. Jan. 20, 2005. http://www.livescience.com/health/050120_brain_sex.html

[39] Gurian, M. (2001). 'Boys and girls learn differently!: A guide for teachers and parents'. San Fransico, CA: Jossey-Bass., page 27

[40] Grey, Dr. John, 'The Male vs. the Female Brain', ThirdAge.com, April 27, 2011, http://www.thirdage.com/love-romance/the-male-vs-the-female-brain

were shown to have potentially more grey matter, more deeply focused thinking, more use of the rational frontal lobe. What amazing advantages!"

I was also intrigued by the concept that some of us on the spectrum (a percentage) are less affected by the emotional reactions triggered in the amygdala; i.e., the primitive fight-or-flight, emotional rushes that stem from the inner reptilian part of our brain and cause us to act before our rational brain can process the information.

I know that in the history of mankind, these types of rapid, emotionally fueled responses have probably been helpful for our survival. If you stand there contemplating possible solutions when a lion is chasing you, you may not live long enough to pass that rational brain on! So back then, it was good that we had a mechanism to let us act without thinking. But is acting without thinking in today's society really an advantage anymore?

I don't exactly need to prepare myself to fight or flee from my boss during a feedback session or from a spouse who has left the toilet seat up. (Well, okay, fleeing from my boss might feel good in the moment, but it wouldn't really help me in the long run.) So wouldn't it just be better if we were able to perhaps feel the emotions but react calmly and rationally at all times anyway? You think that sounds impossible? Well, I know it can happen, because that's exactly how I am, and I think it's an amazing step forward.

But anyway, before I get carried away and "Aspie" you with details, the main thing I want you to take away from the table is how Autism and Asperger's are real brain conditions caused by real neurobiological differences and aren't just a set of "problematic behaviors," as it might seem. The condition causes both positive and negative qualities in a person and can produce some incredibly talented, intelligent, rational, and outside-the-box thinkers. However, we often have trouble interfacing with the typical world.

I wish I could say that the upsides of Autism and Asperger's were well known and understood by the community, but I think in this area, there's still a lot of work to be done. Some people are still afraid of the Autism spectrum and seeking a cure. That's understandable, I guess, if you're caring for and worried about the future for someone on the low-functioning end. But at my end—heavens!—I don't want to be cured! I want to be accommodated and embraced and my "type" encouraged. We need to let people know that Autism has some great sides to it too.

I suppose that historically, doctors and specialists in the area had to be focused on the negatives, because their job is to look for areas in which people may struggle and need help. And so, a lot of the documents out there may just list the negatives. But please always read those documents with that in mind. And remember:

"Autism is not a processing error. It's a different operating system."—Some random flyer that went around Facebook.

What a great analogy.

At any rate, I'll now leave you with the DSM-IV psychological definition of As-perger's Syndrome[42] so you can read through the official symptoms for yourself, but do keep in mind—again—that this is a diagnosis based on *difficulties* only.

DSM-IV definition for Asperger's Syndrome (299.80)[43]

(I)   Qualitative impairment in social interaction, as manifested by at least two of the following:

(A) marked impairments in the use of multiple nonverbal be-haviors such as eye-to-eye gaze, facial expression, body posture, & gestures to regulate social interaction

(B) failure to develop peer relationships appropriate to de-velopmental level

(C) a lack of spontaneous seeking to share enjoyment, inter-ests, or achievements with other people, (e.g. by a lack of showing, bringing, or pointing out objects of interest to other people)

(D) lack of social or emotional reciprocity

(II)   Restricted, repetitive, & stereotyped patterns of behavior, interests, & activities, as manifested by at least one of the following:

(A) encompassing preoccupation with one or more stereo-typed & restricted patterns of interest that is abnormal either in intensity or focus

(B) apparently inflexible adherence to specific, nonfunction-al routines or rituals

(C) stereotyped & repetitive motor mannerisms (e.g. hand or finger flapping or twisting or complex whole-body movements)

---

[42] Note that in May 2013 the DSM IV was updated to the DSM V in which Asperger's was reclassi-fied as part of the Autism spectrum. In the chapter, however, I've chosen to keep the DSM IV defini-tions as I think they do a better job of describing Asperger's specifically.

[43] *Diagnostic and Statistical Manual of Mental Disorders* (4th ed., pp. 70-71) Washington, DC: American Psychiatric Association, 1994

(D) persistent preoccupation with parts of objects

(III)   The disturbance causes clinically significant impairments in social, occupational, or other important areas of functioning.

(IV)   There is no clinically significant general delay in language (e.g. single words used by age 2 years, communicative phrases used by age 3 years).

(V)   There is no clinically significant delay in cognitive development or in the development of age-appropriate self-help skills, adaptive behavior (other than in social interaction), & curiosity about the environment in childhood.

(VI)   Criteria are not met for another specific Pervasive Developmental Disorder or Schizophrenia.

CHAPTER THIRTY-SIX

MOVING TO HOUSTON, TEXAS

And now for the beginning of my adventure overseas.

When Robert first told me that he wanted us to pack up and relocate to Houston, I was quite taken aback and felt strongly against the idea. We'd recently just settled into life in Ormond with a new baby, and I was enjoying my new life and finding my feet. I had my nursery all set up—my perfect little baby place. What do you mean I should take it apart and pack it all up?

But it had become clear that Robert's career was going to require some overseas experience for advancement, and I knew this Houston job offer he'd received was a great opportunity for him. If it wasn't Houston, Robert explained, then it could be Angola, Chad, Qatar, or elsewhere. So, under pressure not to hold him back, I agreed to make a go of it. After all, in comparison to Chad, Houston didn't sound so bad, I reasoned. And it was only a two-to-three-year project. So I decided to think of it as a holiday adventure.

Once the decision was made, I quickly went online and made myself busy investigating this new place—Houston, Texas—that I knew so little about. When I Googled Houston information, the first thing that came up was a pie chart of the population by race—approximately 40 percent Caucasian, 32 percent Hispanic, 16 percent African American, 12 percent Asian or other specific races, and less than 1 percent "mixed." That was odd. I wondered why race should be of concern to anyone and why there was so little interracial mixing. I hadn't lived in a country where there was racial segregation before. I didn't understand it.

The next thing that came up was the weather, typically forty to ninety-five degrees Fahrenheit and twenty-nine to ninety-nine degrees Fahrenheit on the extremes. That didn't sound so bad. I had yet to learn that the Houston summer lasts for almost six months of the year and is relentlessly consistent between ninety and one hundred degrees every day with extreme humidity. It wasn't like Melbourne, where those high temperatures are reached for around five days a year, tempered with the dryness of the heat.

I questioned Robert on how his work would be helping me settle in and was assured that they would find me a local mums' group and activities for the kids. We would have hotel accommodation paid for us for the first month's stay and a relocation consultant to help us with all the transitions and paperwork. I was also told about an active expatriate wives' group which I would be included in. So far, so good. His work seemed very accommodating.

In my head, I pictured this mums' group as a friendly social community of women who hung out together daily, somewhat like compound life but with full access to the greater community. My vision had all the ladies living in their own houses, but right by one another where we could meet up in the mornings to do daily activities with the group—shopping together, going out to parks, and raising the kids together. Perhaps even cooking together or going to each other's houses for the evenings. A place of harmony and warmth.

The concept of living so closely appealed to me in the same way that high school had. Being constantly around others is an easy way for me to make friends—whether they like it or not! I feel secure when I run into the same people every day. It keeps me up to date on their lives and them on mine so I can relax and be me without the need for small talk to bring people up to speed. And if I do say something that goes down badly, I can always be reassured that I'll still see them the next day and the next until it eventually blows over! You know, being stuck in people's faces is a good thing! At least that's what I thought. But it turned out my daydreams were very off the mark.

My friends at home began to stir[44] me about rodeos, cowboy hats, and people saying "y'all" to the crowd. (I was later told in Texas—jokingly—that "y'all" is singular and "all y'all" is the plural!) I saw a clip on TV of a Texan police officer pulling over a car, patting down the driver, and talking to them very seriously. The officer was wearing a khaki-color sheriff's outfit with a badge, a wide-brimmed hat, and a gun in his belt. All humor would've been lost on him! It was down to business. And I thought, "My gosh, where on Earth am I going?"

---

[44] Stir = playfully tease

But there was no time for questioning. The move was pushed through in a great rush. We first heard about the transfer offer in November, and by mid-January, we were on a plane with all our furniture packed up in a ship in the middle of the Pacific Ocean. We would have to survive for a few months on the little we had fit into air freight. And when you consider the immediate needs of a young baby, this was not a lot! Isaac was only four months old at the time of the move.

Settling in our hotel in Houston, rather abruptly, I found myself in for some culture shock in little, unexpected ways. Robert had put some thought into the transition and had selected a hotel by the Galleria so we could be right by shops and buy groceries and everyday needs within walking distance. But amusingly, the Galleria didn't sell groceries! It was an American-style mall, and I'd been clueless about what that meant.

In my hotel room, I couldn't find a kettle to prepare boiled water for the baby bottles the way I was accustomed to. How do people prepare bottles quickly without instant, sterile water on hand, I wondered. When I called the hotel desk to order one, the lady I spoke to didn't seem to know what a "kittle" was but suggested I boil water in a pot on the stove. So that wasn't helpful. And so on it went, with many strange little things that were done differently from what I'd been used to.

Then, just a week or two into the stay, we had the most awful experience, which ended up with Isaac in the hospital overnight. Unbeknownst to me, Isaac was intolerant to the American formula we changed to and, over the course of a week, started vomiting up to several times a day. I assumed he'd picked up a local cold that one of his little friends was suffering from, so I let it go a day or two. Robert had already commenced work, so I was attending him alone, unable to drive yet. But one afternoon, Isaac cried so intensely that I called Robert to come home and we rushed to the emergency room.

Isaac ended up put on an IV for dehydration and was sent in an ambulance to Texas Children's Hospital. In an unfamiliar country, it was terrifying. I can't even describe to you the horror of being a new mother holding your little baby limp in your arms. Thankfully, the hospital was able to identify his problem as milk protein intolerance and set us up with the right formula, and he remained healthy from then on.

But despite that awful bit of initial drama, I felt positive overall about the move and started to find my feet quickly.

After I'd been at the hotel a few weeks, another expatriate mum, Carina, came and joined me with her two-year-old son. Our husbands had moved role at similar times and had organized for us to stay at the same hotel. It was a big relief to me to have someone to cling to (don't tell her I worded it that way!), and we got along well and quickly began the process of navigating Houston together—or perhaps the truth is that she led me.

Carina showed me the way to the local grocery store, and we would walk our strollers down together to pick up supplies. I went to her hotel room one day, and we lay on her bed talking about real estate and where we planned to move.

During our various wandering, Carina often would get phone calls regarding various elements of her move that would delay our walks significantly. I myself had avoided getting a phone and having to call people. I left most of that sort of organizing to my husband, so I was unstressed and at my leisure. But despite her occasional busyness, we did end up with a lot of free one-on-one time. We talked about most things that two ladies might talk about.

Over the same time period, I also found out that the local Houston expatriate wives met up every Friday at a café, and I was invited to join them. I wanted to go, but driving on the other side of the road was daunting at first (we drive on the left in Australia), and I took a while to ease into it. So it was some months before I was mobile enough to get myself there. Carina seemed quite confident in the car and had jumped straight into driving around. She gave me a lift to the café once, and that was the first time that I met the other ladies. For me, it was an uncomfortable group of strangers, but at least they seemed welcoming.

Around a month after arriving, Carina and her family moved on to their rental house in the far north of Houston, and I found a rental downtown at least an hour away. The house search process had been rapid, as we'd had a limited period in which the company covered hotel expenses. We settled for a house in a wealthy, green-treed, "inner-loop" area near my husband's work.

The presentation of the area was flawless—the gardens manicured and seamless, the houses freshly painted and swept and set toward the back of the blocks to show off the large front yards. Many front windows were without curtains, allowing viewing of a finely furnished "show-off room" to the street.

We found out, upon touring the house, that our landlords had lowered the price to attract the right tenants, and they took to us with our young baby. So we got a pretty good deal.

Upon moving out of the hotel, I remember feeling a great sense of relief at finally getting away from the room service and having private space to myself. I know it probably sounds odd that I would want help to go away, but as an introvert, I just liked my private space!

Moving into my new house, the neighborhood seemed serene and friendly at first, and I was relieved to discover how safe it was. I'd been concerned about living in a place where people carry guns and crime statistics per unit population were high. But the Houston police were everywhere, driving patrol cars past our front yard every hour or so, directing traffic, or even sitting on motorcycles by the front door. I guess the crime wasn't in our area!

Seeing so many policemen was sometimes unnerving, certainly something that would seem unnecessary at home. But I got used to their presence and stopped noticing surprisingly quickly. It's disconcerting, really, how quickly we just accept the status quo.

However, after a few months of living on our street, my impressions changed, and the neighborhood started to feel more empty and superficial. When I took Isaac for a walk down the streets, I would encounter maids, gardeners, and nannies with children, but few of the property residents.

The children were almost always Caucasian with Hispanic carers, which just struck me as different. In theory, it should've all been fine regardless, but here, there was a language barrier, and I quickly got a sense that me joining in socially with the child-care people just wasn't going to come across as normal. It was a situation that felt awkward, and I didn't know what to do about it.

I found out that the other locals who lived on the same street were usually "busy" out and about (doing who knows what). I met a lovely lady who lived across the road from us. She cooed over Isaac and expressed enthusiasm about coming to visit him regularly, but each time I tried to organize it, she had to cancel on me. One time, her church suddenly needed her at the last minute. Another time, she had to drive a friend's daughter to a funeral. And so it went.

In the end, I realized she was just too busy and heavily leaned upon by others, and I gave up. The neighbor to the side talked about hosting a small gathering to welcome me into the street, which would have been perfect, but she also never found the time to make it happen.

I soon learnt that it was the American or at least Houston culture to greet others with great enthusiasm and talk about catch-ups and doing things together but not always follow through. At home, this would be considered a little rude. But here, I guess it was the social ritual. A similar ritual to saying, "Hi, how are you?" "Let's catch up some time." A polite line with no meaning. And the people here are just used to knowing that it's all talk.

I also learnt that it was the culture for people to rush from place to place. Somebody will come over for a dinner and then have to leave because they have another dinner to go to. Multiple events would be planned for single afternoons or evenings. What a crazy, hectic lifestyle.

This part of the culture didn't suit me well, as I personally take a while to relax and settle in to a social occasion. When I see friends, I like to take my time with them and talk to them properly over hours. Such is the culture at home. But it wasn't the Houston way.

In the end, I never did manage to make more than acquaintances of any of the neighbors. They were interested in smiling and having keen, welcoming, nice-to-see-you chats on the odd occasions when I ran into them, but I didn't get any further than that. I wonder if it would have been the same had I moved into a less wealthy suburb.

I asked the relocation consultant that Robert's work had assigned us about mums' groups in the area. At home, the local child help centers would gather people with babies of the same age to attend training together on raising a child and for social gathering. Playgroups Australia will also organize for local playgroups for children of similar age. I was told that there was nothing like that here, only the private gatherings that individuals might happen to organize. She was unable to locate any near my area.

At the same time, I began going to the weekly Houston expatriate wives' meetups. Carina had moved too far away to be involved in these, but I met a lot of other seemingly nice ladies, and initially, things appeared to be going well. I would take Isaac to the café, and he would play with the other children while I sat, ate lunch, and talked.

It was a large group, so I didn't get much opportunity to go into more juicy topics, but I was doing okay with the small talk, or at least I seemed to be acting the part well. I can't say it was exactly stimulating for me. Besides, initially, I was so busy setting up house that I didn't mind the large portions of time by myself in between.

But then, time passed and nothing changed . . . and more time passed again and nothing changed . . . and yet more time again . . . and after many months of sameness, it occurred to me that I wasn't getting anywhere with making friends. With so much time alone each week, I was starting to get bored, and boredom can be depressing.

Looking at the other ladies around me, I could see that they were interacting. Outside of the group, they were going over to each other's houses for coffee and dinners or ringing each other up about events that were on to make spur-of-the-moment arrangements. There would be little chats about it here and there at the café meetup. How much fun people had had at little things here and there that I hadn't heard of or been invited to. I started to wonder why I wasn't falling into these smaller social circles too.

It became clear that what I needed to do was make some closer friends. But how? How do I get involved in real conversations with people in such an Aspie-unfriendly large group setting?

Back at school and university, it wasn't so hard to meet people in more private situations, because, love me or hate me, every day we would have to be there in the common room together! But here, time spent together was spontaneous and completely voluntary, and I had no idea how to break in.

I lamented about how nice it would have been to have that imaginary expat community I'd dreamed up when I first envisioned coming to Houston—the fun communal living situation I'd imagined, like the one that Carina and I had had. No rallying to be on the invite list or calling around to see what's on. Just an automatic invite to whatever routine thing was on, day in, day out, with the same people every time. It seemed the obvious way to do things to me. Why couldn't real life be simple like this? But I guess it wasn't the way the expat ladies wanted to do it out here in the great U. S. of A. Real life was complicated.

I was a straggler in the group, and I didn't know what to do about it. And things only got harder from there.

To be continued . . .

CHAPTER THIRTY-SEVEN

ASPERGER'S AND BEING A MUM

Q: Is it difficult having Asperger's Syndrome and being a mother? Do you feel you're adequate/good as a parent?

Ah, yes. The parenting question. I'd been expecting that one!

The question of whether I, as an Aspie, could be an adequate parent rather shocks me and scares me at the same time. It brings to my mind fearful concepts like eugenics or someone proposing the removal of children from disabled parents to give them a "proper" upbringing, not unlike some scary times in history, such as the lost generation of Aborigines in Australia. Fortunately, I don't live in a world where any of that is likely to happen, but it is an awful thought nonetheless.

I know that, as a parent, I've *always* been incredibly loving, and anybody who sees me with my children would agree. The emotions I hold for my boys are so strong, they overwhelm me at times, and if anything, it makes me a more protective and thoughtful parent than most, always analyzing what is best for my children's long-term well-being.

As a person, I'm warm and kind and tend to be good at bonding with children, as unexpected as that may seem. In fact, I hear that it's not uncommon for Aspies to be intuitively good with children and/or animals, at least for those of us who take an interest! I think it's because we don't hide behind pretend enthusiasm and vocal inflection.

When we feel affection, we show it openly in our physical language, even without specifically meaning to, and this transparency makes kids and pets feel safe around us.

When working in the childcare scene some years back, I had colleagues comment that I was quick to win over insecure children and especially popular with those who needed that little extra attention or calming. I know it sounds odd, given my natural difficulties with social interactions, but children aren't difficult to read the way adults can be.

As a parent myself, I've been fortunate to find myself able to understand my oldest son—who has some rather strong Aspie traits of his own—well, and I'm so glad that I'm the one raising him. I'm in the right position to give him the understanding and positive encouragement that he needs, and it makes me so sad to imagine how he might have fared growing up in a family that just couldn't make sense of him the same way. He's my darling. My angel. My sweetest little boy, and I want the world for him.

Of course, having said all that, that doesn't mean that parenting is *easy* for me. Like the rest of you, I'm continually battling with that grey area that is child rearing: knowing how to respond to each situation and trying to figure out which demands are reasonable and which are not, juggling the constant needs and wants of two children always both vying for my attention at the same time, and trying not to go insane over the unbelievable tantrums they will throw over things like, "I didn't want to wee. Put the wee back in me! PUT THE WEE BACK INNNNN!!!"

And on top of the usual, with this Aspie brain of mine, I also seem to have a few other troubles which are more unique to me individually.

For example, being on the spectrum, it's natural for me to want to have periods where I block everything out and become absorbed in the project at hand whenever the inspiration takes me, or sometimes when I just need a break to calm down from being overstimulated or overanxious. I'm wired to want to intensely focus on a subject and just live there for a while, so interruptions can become intolerable at those times. However, with a two-year-old around, life is a barrage of interruptions!

Early on, I noticed my tendency to become crabby at the times when I used to try and focus on "my things" and my older son would come up wanting to talk to me, so I've had to make up rules for myself to keep my behavior in check, like no writing when Isaac is around and no editing photographs when Isaac is around. Basically, no doing anything that draws my focus too much. By following these rules, I've been able to keep my parenting mostly calm and positive, and I'm proud of myself for this. However, it does take a toll on me and a lot of self-control on my part. And boy, does it limit how much I can get done in a day!

Sometimes I feel frustrated about tasks niggling at me in the back of my mind. I get caught up imagining what I want to do or say when I get a chance and find myself tuning out of real life a little too easily!

However, I keep reminding myself that parenting the boys in a kind and tolerant way is critical for their self-esteem, and I want them to grow up confident and happy, which is much more important than any little task I want to do. So this frustration is something I'm just going to have to accept for the next few years until they're old enough to both be in school. (Hooray for that day! I mean, aww, I'll miss them.)

In the meanwhile, I do get some relief by putting Isaac in a mother's day out program two mornings a week or hiring a lady to come and take him to the park from time to time. So this has afforded me most of the time I've used to get this writing done and thankfully kept me sane!

As an Aspie mum, I've also noticed that trying to socialize in playgroup-type settings can be pretty rough on me. If you remember, I'm not wired for multitasking, so I get a bit lost trying to watch both of the boys and interact with the adults at the same time. My focus is either on one or the other or, at best, jumping back and forth between the two, which is confusing for me. Even keeping up with "typical" adults alone can be hard enough!

Sometimes, out at a park with the mums and kids and noise and light and chaos everywhere, it becomes too exhausting and I end up retreating to just following my kids around and interacting only with them. I'm sure this looks antisocial or aloof to other mums, and maybe they take it badly, but if I've reached this point, then it means I'm too tired or exasperated to keep trying. It's my fallback, especially in public places where the noise and light alone is sometimes all I can deal with. I'm sure the other mums think I'm a little strange.

When my first son, Isaac, was about one, I actually had another expat mum (Angel) point this difficulty out to me. She said she noticed how distracted I get when Isaac comes up and talks to me and how I lose my place in the conversation. On the surface, it's subtle to see, but obviously, it was visible enough for her to notice.

When she said it, it surprised me at first, because I hadn't fully realized that other mothers don't have the same difficulty. But observing other mums, I see now that they jump between talking to each other and directing/responding to the kids with ease. It doesn't distract them from the discussion being had. I guess that's an ability I just don't have.

Building on this thought, I had an incident in the mall just recently that showed me how much I ignore other adults when I'm focusing on the boys, and it surprised me, because I wasn't really aware of the extent to which I do that. I thought I was good at picking up signals, but I suppose to pick them up, I have to be actively looking for them.

I was sitting at the mall playground with a good friend of mine, Josh, when my baby son, Trent, crawled up and started cooing and grabbing at a lady on one of the seats. At first, she was happy to smile and talk to him, commenting to me how cute he was. I saw that Trent was getting a lot of positive attention, so I happily moved on to talking to Josh and keeping an ear out for the boys.

A minute or so later, Josh commented to me that he thought the lady had had enough of Trent now. I looked over at her and sure enough, she was facing away from him and blocking him out. Trent was still cooing and happy, so I hadn't picked it up! I went over and picked him up to move him away. As I did, the lady smiled and said to me, "Oh, he is so cute," in a bubbly tone. It confused me. I thought, "Oh, do you want me to give him back so he can play some more?" I wasn't sure, so I took him with me.

When I sat back down, Josh told me that he thought, "Oh, he is so cute," meant, "Thank you for taking him away," and I realized that he was right. Instead of politely saying to me, "I've had enough now. Can you please take your baby?" the lady had used body language to signal it while saying exactly the opposite with her words.

This is frustrating to me, because if I don't look for the signals, I can completely miss the meaning. Having a friend with me to explain things was a novelty, and it surprised me a few times to hear what he'd picked up that I hadn't. It makes me wonder how many other communications I haven't seen over time. Perhaps it might explain why sometimes mums go hot and cold with me for no apparent reason. If I'm not looking out for their subtle hints, then I may not understand what they want from me until they get angry. It's no wonder I'd been finding the mums' groups so difficult.

But, of course, none of these little issues make me in any way unsuitable as a parent, and I'm not implying that I'm not up for the job. I have my challenges, but the boys don't suffer for them. We maintain a warm, close, loving relationship in a way that I'm starting to think is very special and rare.

I lay on the floor with Isaac, and we cuddle and play tickling games. He covers me with face washers[45] from the kitchen cupboard and rearranges my hair. I crawl around the room after him pretending to be a crocodile, and he yells, "No, Mummy, don't be scary," and then, "Again." He makes an imaginary castle out of his sleeping mat, and we hide in it together. We roughhouse like boys do.

I love watching him be sweet with his little brother. He gives him toys and hugs and kisses. I hear Isaac yelling boo from the back seat of the car when I'm driving, and Trent giggles and coos from his capsule.[46]

When I place Isaac in the care of others, I'm extra cautious to make sure of the quality of care. I've experienced the negative impact of bullying myself, and I'm proactive about making sure he doesn't experience any belittling. I know Isaac has challenging behaviors—a likely Aspie himself, I think—and I get involved to make sure

---

[45] Face washers = washcloths

[46] Capsule = a detachable-style infant car seat

the teachers are redirecting him positively and not misunderstanding him. I pay close attention to how he's responding to the school experience.

I think part of what makes me a good mum is that I don't fall into the trap of being too focused on controlling my kids and worrying about how we appear to others. I know I can't let them get too unruly or they'll irritate people, but I tend to draw that line closer to the side of what is in the best interests of the boys, not based on who is frowning at me or who wants me to do it their way.

One big upside to being an Aspie is that no matter how emotional the kids make me, I can always think logically about what I'm doing and the long-term impact it'll have on them. So I adjust my behavior accordingly and spend a lot of time thinking about my parenting techniques and how the boys are coming along.

I know some people wonder if an Aspie can be empathetic and in tune enough with a child to respond appropriately with empathy and affection, but you know, you don't need to pick up everything to be a caring, compassionate parent. I love my boys, and they know they're loved. I give them lots of cuddles, words of praise, and physical affection (patting, tickling, etc.). They smile and laugh with me frequently. I respond to them and comfort them when they're unhappy. I think these are the things that really count.

CHAPTER THIRTY-EIGHT

DOING THINGS AND DOING THEM "RIGHT"

Okay, now time for another one of those ad hoc trains of thought that just wandered into my head . . .

In one of my early League meetings, I remember a fellow Aspie quoting the line, "If something is worth doing, it's worth doing right." And I don't know why I was lying in bed thinking about that now, but I decided to bring it up because I think that is a very Aspie philosophy and a common trait among many of us. When we are passionate enough to want to do something, we want it done well. The goal isn't just to get it done but to achieve something to be proud of. Often, we go above and beyond expectations if that's what it takes to meet our vision. Aspies excel at doing exceptional things!

I myself have always been a little bothered by sloppiness, inaccuracies in calculations, numbers not adding up, or messy or inconsistent presentation. I just have this itch to want things correct, consistent, and in their proper place. Ah, no—all those lines are indented but that one. I can't handle that!

Call it meticulous, but it's the perfectionist in me, and I don't feel satisfied with my work until I've achieved this. I suppose the big difference between Autistic people and typical people is that we are task focused and all about doing the task right, whereas neurotypicals are usually more impression focused and concerned more about how their work appears to others.

I recall one of the League members, Rob, once commenting that everything he's done, job or hobby, he's always been exceptionally good at, a stand-out talent. And while people reading those words might assume it's arrogance, I have to say I also relate to the feeling of being naturally strong at anything I put my mind to. It seems to be the case for those of us who share this perfectionist trait. We excel because we take so much pride in what we do. Combining this with Aspie hyperfocus allows us to outdo what most can achieve. We become visionary.

Unfortunately, I've seen that not all working roles are suited to this type of focus and perfection. Some places put more emphasis on producing rapidly and cheaply and may prefer staff to work faster, even if to a lower standard. Some are more focused on politics and appearances than actual quality of work, and we can be out of place in these environments.

However, I think there are many roles that could really take advantage of our scrupulous nature, and in fact, I read recently a report about some companies seeking people on the spectrum for this very reason. I think that's a terrific step forward for the Autistic community.

It would be nice if, in time, society could come to recognize us more for the things we *can* do and stop seeing us as a drain when we struggle to work and make money in the standard way. Though our culture teaches us otherwise, working nine to five is not the only way to give back to the world. You should see what some of us contribute in our hobbies! We are anything but a drain on the community at large. On the contrary, as a group, paid or unpaid, we create a lot!

And I know that's a point I've probably made before, but I think it's worth repeating. We Aspies can help society a lot if you only accommodate us. Accommodate us, world! I'm telling you, it's worth it!

Chapter Thirty-Nine

Being Diagnosed with Asperger's Syndrome

And now, digging back into the heart of my Aspie journey:

Q: How did you find out you have Asperger's Syndrome, and what was it like to get diagnosed?

Ah, yes. Coming to understand about my Asperger's and then being diagnosed with it was a very, *very* strange thing for me.

Growing up, as you know, I'd never even heard of the word Asperger's, let alone had any notion of what it was or that I, of all people, could have such a "syndrome." A label on me sounded ridiculous. I was highly intelligent, logical, and capable of achieving in ways above and beyond what most people can achieve. I felt more like someone extraordinary or exemplary than someone with a "syndrome." So, as you can imagine, this discovery process has been a rapid learning experience for me over the last five or so years.

I first heard of the term Asperger's when I was around twenty-seven, while hanging out with Girls' Group at one of their weekly gatherings. The group was having a discussion in which we were given questions to prompt us to talk about our life experiences and how we handle particular situations. I can't remember the specific topic now, but something about my inner Aspie must have come out, because my friend Emma, now a child psychologist, asked me if I'd ever heard of Asperger's Syndrome.

I remember after she told me briefly about it, she picked up a coffee cup and said, "Raaa, I'm a dinosaur. I'm going to get you," (or something like that) advancing the cup on me. It was a test to see how literally I would take it. As a child, perhaps I wouldn't have found it funny and would have told her flatly, "That's not a dinosaur. It's a cup." But as an adult who is well versed in working with kids, I understand pretend play and appreciate a quirky sense of humor. So I laughed at the bizarre gesture and just said, "Okay, sure. It's a dinosaur."

We didn't decide one way or another that night whether we thought I really had Asperger's, but Emma had explained it a little and planted the seed in my head. (Not literally!) I walked away thinking perhaps I might have a "little bit" of it. It would explain a lot of things. But I didn't take it too seriously. After all, the way she'd described it was more textbook Asperger's, and I felt far more adapted than that.

Not too long after this discussion, I looked up Asperger's Syndrome on the internet and found the DSM-IV definition and some general information on the topic. But what I read sounded serious: descriptions of people with a debilitating behavioral disorder. I thought, "Well, that doesn't describe me. I'm 'normal.' Perhaps I share some of these traits, but I'm not severely disabled or ignorant on how to act around others. This is not me." So I closed the book on the subject and didn't revisit it for several years. And that was that.

Then one day, quite a few years later, long after I'd ceased ever thinking about the topic, I remember sitting in my house in Houston, really struggling with the isolation and boredom that had come from moving to a place where I was failing to establish solid friends. This is the place where I left off in the last story chapter.

I was trying to watch TV and turned on a psychological reality series called *The OCD Project*, a show where the participants lived together in a house and were counseled to overcome their various OCDs, when strangely, one of the participants, a man diagnosed with Asperger's during the series, got me thinking again about the possibility of having Asperger's myself.

The way it triggered the thought was a little odd, because the man was nothing like me at all. He was extremely unusual in his mannerisms and had trouble understanding and accepting some simple concepts and tasks. He had satanic delusions and severe OCD. If anything, seeing this character should have perpetuated my notion that people with Asperger's are "weird" and that I couldn't be one of them. But something he did resonated with me, and it resonated strongly. It was something about the way he resisted emotional counseling.

It took me back to a time a few years earlier when I'd tried to go to a counselor myself to see if they could help with work and social issues. I remember explaining to the man I saw that, "While I function well on the surface, I know underneath, I battle with the need to constantly analyze to work out what people are thinking of me and respond appropriately, and social interactions are exhausting and sometimes stressful."

I'd come up with a theory that maybe I had social anxiety, which may have been true to some degree back then, but I'm sure nowhere near as severely as my Asperger's makes it seem. I was hoping that if a counselor could make it "go away," then perhaps work and large social situations could become comfortable and bearable for me.

The counselor got me to take a few social anxiety quizzes, and from his responses, I think he concluded I had notable social anxiety, although I think half of what he was picking up was my Asperger's tendencies and the side effects of those.

With questions like, "Do you ever feel overwhelmed or 'stressed out?' Do you ever fear that you will do or say the wrong thing in front of other people? Do you feel trapped in or avoid social situations where it might be difficult to escape, such as in a crowd? Do you ever push yourself to do more, even when you're physically and mentally exhausted?"—it's hard not to mistake some of the Asperger's traits for anxiety if anxiety is all you're testing for. There is a huge overlap.

After the testing, he then went on to "treat" me with a range of exercises that somehow seemed to only frustrate and tire me. He asked me to make lists showing each time I had negative feelings for a week and describe the self-talk behind each feeling. I didn't know what to write down. I knew when I was starting to have negative emotions but not how to identify the emotion or what was causing it. It usually just stems from exhaustion, overstimulation, and/or frustration slowly building up. (I know that now.)

I wrote down a few thoughts that were very minor, because I felt like I had to do the homework and write something. It was almost like making it up. I really didn't have any negative self-talk that I dwelled on. He then made a big fuss over each thing I wrote down and wanted to dig deeper into the emotions behind them. All I could say in response was, "I don't know," and, "No, not really." I felt tired of it and resistant. I wanted to tell him, "Stop wasting my time with this crap."

He asked me to role-play scenarios with him. A tall, lanky man with hairy legs, he would cross his legs and say to pretend he was a female friend and make dialogue with him. I couldn't do it. How could I pretend he was someone he wasn't and then imagine how I would feel in the situation? I couldn't formulate a realistic response, because I had no idea how I would feel if a real woman said these things to me.

The ridiculousness of him trying to act the role made me want to laugh and unable to take it seriously. He had hairy legs for heaven's sakes! He told me to try. I felt like a child being scolded. His insistence I "try" when I just couldn't imagine the scenario upset me and made me feel belittled. All I could see was a big, hairy man with his legs crossed like a woman being stern with me. I wanted to laugh and then cry as my laughter was frowned upon.

And so it went on for six sessions, exercise after exercise that were all similarly ineffective and frustrating for me. I found myself not wanting to go and starting to feel hostile toward him. This reaction surprised me, because I'd come to him genuinely wanting to learn, and I'm usually fascinated about psychology and learning about my brain. I'm an obedient type who does my homework, not the type who rebels and defies the teacher. Yet here I was, becoming increasingly frustrated and resistant.

After the six sessions were up, I told him I wasn't comfortable with a male and wanted to transfer to another counselor—a neurotypical-style white lie—so he gave me a reference and wished me well. Of course, I never went. I decided by this point that I was better equipped to deal with my own issues than waste money on exercises I was only going to resist. I gave up the idea of seeing a counselor at all. After all, I think I do a good job of finding the right balance for me on how hard to push myself. So I decided I didn't need to do tiring exercises to achieve this.

In a way, I was lucky that my counseling experience was by choice and I had the right to walk away. I wonder how many poor teens are placed into such counseling by parents and loved ones only to be forced to try and do things they can't do and made to feel "bad" or rebellious for not taking it seriously or not trying. I can see how it would be incredibly deflating.

Coming back to the point in time where I was watching *The OCD Project*, I was amazed to see another man having the same responses to the counseling that I'd had. I watched him try and argue logically why the exercises were a waste of time or try to alter them to make them work for him only to be told to "just try it." The counseling was based on emotions, not logic or theory, and it simply wasn't hitting home.

When I saw him removed from the series and diagnosed with Asperger's, the lightbulb suddenly came on for me. Maybe I have Asperger's too. Maybe that's why all this emotional crap felt pointless and impossible for me to do: it's not tailored to a brain like my own.

After that realization, I went immediately to the computer—mid-episode, in fact—and started researching Asperger's again. It was a moment of sudden fascination. I needed to know. This time, I found forums and discussions by real people with real Asperger's experiences, not just behavioral summaries written from neurotypical perspectives. The real Aspies were *not* saying:

- "I have impairments in nonverbal behaviors such as eye-to-eye gaze, facial expression, body posture, and gestures to regulate social interaction."
- "I lack social or emotional reciprocity."
- "I show apparently inflexible adherence to specific, nonfunctional routines or rituals."

They were saying things like:

- "I hate having to go to big social functions. I like small groups."
- "I never know when to cut into the conversation."
- "Other people don't seem to like deep conversations the way I do."
- "Once people really get to know me, they seem to lose interest in hanging out with me for no obvious reason."
- "I'm tired of having to work so hard to do and say the right thing all the time."
- "People get offended for no reason."

The more I read, the more I realized this really is me! I joined one of the forums and became an active participant and began to learn more and more about what Asperger's really means.

A few months after this initial discovery, I decided to seek the counsel of a psychologist for a professional diagnosis.

The decision to have myself diagnosed wasn't one I made easily, and reading online, I saw a lot of warning against it. People were warning of being forced to reveal the diagnosis when applying for jobs and being discriminated against for it. They were saying it doesn't help socially to have a label. And, of course, there's the fact that it doesn't actually change who you are. With or without diagnosis, you are still the person you were yesterday, so why do you need it?

However, I reasoned that I was never going to be okay in a job where I had to suppress my Asperger's. My past experiences have showed me that it is not sustainable for me to work the typical way. If I ever did apply for a job again, it would have to be with full disclosure so that I could have the necessary accommodations made for me and the political expectations of me be more realistic.

As for friends, I could always choose whether I wished to tell them or not. There's no requirement there, and if anything, having a formal diagnosis could only help in terms of getting relatives or skeptics to believe me. Though it turns out that getting people to believe me has been no problem. Most people I've told have responded with comments such as, "Ah, that makes sense!"

Mostly, however, I sought diagnosis because something inside me just needed to know for sure. As irrational and "unlike an Aspie" as that sounds, there was a strong emotional driver there for me to know myself and be validated. I felt as if I couldn't rest until I knew. So with no strong reason not to get diagnosed, I yielded to that feeling. And for one of the few times in my life, I made a purely emotional decision.

Upon selecting a counselor, I was careful to look for someone who had knowledge of adult Asperger's Syndrome. It turned out this was a tricky thing to find, as most experts seem to specialize in children. Online, I was reading that even those who are experts in childhood Asperger's aren't always good at picking up the more subtle adult form of the condition.

One lady wrote of how she was dismissed without even being tested because a counselor told her she was "too normal to have Asperger's." Another man wrote of how a general practitioner had said to him he couldn't have Asperger's because "people with that syndrome collect shiny metal objects," and he didn't do that. What are we, nesting birds?

However, despite my fears of being turned away for acting the normal role too well, I was eventually directed to a lady who was very experienced in counseling adults and even women with Asperger's, and I had a surprisingly pleasant experience. She didn't just take me at face value. She asked me some deep and detailed questions that showed a real knowledge of where Asperger's really presents itself.

After a short phone interview, I set up my first appointment for the two-stage diagnostic process. Step one was a detailed discussion to understand my background and determine whether Asperger's was likely, and step two was the detailed testing.

My first interview session with the doctor was profound. Though I was new to the idea of having Asperger's, she got me thinking back into my past and realizing so many Asperger's moments I'd forgotten about. So many things started to make sense (i.e., many of the random stories I've presented in this book!). It was like having the biggest realization of my life. In only a few short hours, I was given answers to questions I'd been unable to answer for years.

She explained to me what that feeling was that I'd been getting in the workplace: the buildup of frustration and stress from overstimulation and all the irritating things that I had to suppress and not react to during a typical day. I'd come up with so many possible explanations for it over the years, and none had been even close.

She told me it wasn't the first time she'd heard this story. What an amazing feeling to realize that there are others in the world who have gone through what I have! It was the final validation that it's okay for me to find these things difficult.

I was finally free to say no, I'm not prepared to suffer this way anymore, and I have a valid reason for it. I walked away from the session buzzing with realizations, new thoughts and memories, and the high of feeling like I was finally free. I don't think I slept that night at all.

The second session was simpler. I came in, sat down at a table, and filled out a multitude of tests that the doctor had selected for me. Most of the questions required me to rate on a scale how much I agreed or disagreed with a statement. I found them easy to answer. There were a few short-answer questions that took me longer, basically to establish my history.

Some forms asked for parents or people who knew me growing up to write a few words, but I had nobody to complete these, so I had to guess myself from what I remembered of my childhood. The whole thing took me three or four hours, and then I went home and waited for the results.

After some weeks, the results arrived in the form of a long letter on a company header, detailing my history, the results of the session, and finally stating, "Taken together, these results indicate significant anxiety and depressed mood together with historical and current evidence to support a diagnosis of Asperger's Syndrome." At first, the format of the results threw me. I guess I was expecting a big certificate stating, "Michelle Vines has been diagnosed with (drumroll!) Asperger's Syndrome." I'm not sure why I had this expectation.

The letter I received was more like a discussion containing a lot of personal information. I wrote back to the counselor asking for a shorter version of the diagnosis with less personal information that would be suitable to show a potential employer or anyone else I wished to divulge to.

The doctor obliged and wrote me a short version with the personal information removed, although it did still mention the co-diagnosis of anxiety and depression. I thought, "This will not do. I don't want an employer to read that." But then I thought about it more and realized, who am I going to show anyway?

It's sort of funny that I'd formed an idea I would need to walk in to some situations with documents proving my Asperger's Syndrome, not unlike carrying a visa or a passport! However, employers aren't going to ask me to prove my Asperger's at an interview. What do I need a certificate for? To hang on my wall? Actually, it could be fun to have an Asperger's certificate to hang and be proud of. But I don't need one for any practical purpose.

And then that was it. My formal diagnosis was done. It doesn't change anything for me, but I'm glad to have had it done. It gives me validation and a kind of clarity that comes with really knowing myself, and I was glad to have the opportunity to discuss my Asperger's with a professional and learn the answers to many puzzles that had been plaguing me. I'm glad to know that it's right for me to be the way that I am and that I don't have to justify myself to anyone or pretend to be anything that I'm not.

The more I let the real me come out, the more I grow to like who I am, and I'm finding that others like my charms and quirkiness too. I'm proud of my talents, intellectual abilities, and uniqueness, and I wouldn't want to be anything other than myself. And now that I know the label that comes with that and that there are others like me, I want to wear it with pride and strive to show the rest of the world what a great lot we Aspies are. We are the best! People just need to look past the stereotypes and see it!

Chapter Forty

Areas I Have Difficulty With

Q: So, you function quite well on a day-to-day level. What areas do you find you still have difficulty with?

Ah, yet another good question. I have to say that for an Aspie, I've been pretty lucky.

Through my life experience, I've learnt many little ways to compensate for many of the usual difficulties that Aspies face. Things like taking notes and keeping a diary allow me to function efficiently both at home and at work. Learning detailed social protocol gets me by quite well in the business world and general public eye. I tend to at least appear to fit in and perform well. However, there's one particular area that I continue to have trouble with.

Aside from the obvious issues of coping in the work environment and making neurotypical friends, it's those little chores and tasks that really niggle at me and cause me unreasonable amounts of stress. I'm talking about those "simple" jobs that most people just pick up the phone and deal with as they arise, tasks that require contacting people, finding out information that can't just be looked up online, or having to shop around to find the things I need.

When I drive down the street, my windscreen cracks and needs repair. I notice the car inspection sticker is almost expired and the car will need a new one soon. I pick up my son and there's a note about a theme day coming up that I'm supposed to help provide supplies for. The sign-up sheet asks me to write down what I'll bring. At home, the neighbor comes to the door and suggests that our grass has a brown patch, possibly an infestation that we need to hire a gardener to check out. Every day, there are too many new things to do that I don't know how to start, and it overwhelms me!

Now, I know nobody likes doing chores, but to me, these jobs are something extra. They require social networking and word of mouth. Each one is a brick upon my shoulders to be battled against to stay upright.

For typical people, I think a part of day-to-day life is passing on tips and contact information to each other. Most people easily pick up the details of where to go and what to do to get the day-to-day stuff sorted or whom to ring to find out. But somehow, I just don't.

Ask me about solving simultaneous equations, and I can give you an exciting, detailed answer, but which windshield repair companies in the area are the good ones? That's really not the stuff that sticks in my memory! Tackling a job like this, I'll probably sit and stare at the computer for twenty minutes before I even start, feeling lost as to what to do first and resistant to taking the first step. It's stressful. How do I know whom to trust? Too many of these jobs at a time, and suddenly the bricks are caving in on me!

So who do I hire to fix grass? I don't personally know any specialty gardeners. Our local gardeners just do the standard leaf-blowing, weeding, and trimming service and don't have that sort of expertise. What do I even look up to locate a grass-bug specialist? How many phone calls will it take me to find the right person, and how will I know who is good and who isn't? Are they going to rip me off? Is the problem even caused by bugs? It would be so much easier if there were just someone to tell me who to ring, or—even better—ring them for me! If only I were so lucky!

And why does everything have to require phone calls? As I've mentioned earlier, having to make calls causes me a lot of stress, and I tend to avoid it when I can. I already feel overworked and overstressed most of the time. I don't need additional ringing around to do to add to the load.

Then, when shopping for the kids' party supplies, where do I go to find them? I don't really have that much spare time to spend strolling around shops aimlessly. Shopping is exhausting, and I already have a long backlog of things I need to buy for myself and my kids—a coat for winter, for example! (I get so little kid-free time to do it in as it is.) If I had the additional free shopping time, I'd be buying those things that I need first. Baskets and bonbons are the last thing on my priority list! I'm sorry, but I just can't handle that sign-up list just now. I have too many things to do. I can't deal with this . . .

Stress stress stress stress stress!

Thank heavens I have people in my life to lean on and help me get some of these jobs done. Otherwise, I think I might explode!

So, is this block when it comes to getting things done a problem for all Aspies? I don't think so. I think, like most traits, some of us display it and some don't. I know several Aspies who seem to get through life's chores just fine and at least two others who get similarly overwhelmed to the point of mentally falling apart when it all just gets too much. For me, the stress levels involved can rise so high, they become immobilizing, at least temporarily, until I let go of everything I have to do and calm down. So what should I do about it?

Obviously, the only right solution is that the Aspies who struggle in this way should be assigned our own personal assistant to deal with all this day-to-day crap. I keep saying it! We could push a button that says "NT" to make a person appear and do the paperwork for us and ask them to peel us a grape and fan us with giant palm fronds while we sip cocktails on a deck chair. Then, when their chores were done, we could push another button to dismiss them and give ourselves some quiet time.

Oh dear, I think my editor just had a fit! But, of course, I'm being facetious here. I would never actually degrade a person in that way! It's okay, Hilary. Don't panic. So I guess that idea isn't realistic. Oh well. I guess I'll just have to cope with it the exhausting way then.

Chapter Forty-One

Life in Houston— Expatriate Mums, Part One

Sitting at the playground, I can see a water skimmer, a little fly-like bug perched on the surface of a puddle. I can't really see it moving more than a twitch, but it must be, because it's making little ripples outward intermittently. The moving circles bend the light, and reflections of the sky and tree branches shake before coming steady again. The twigs distort in unusual ways. It's fascinating. I'm watching to see if I can pick up where the little movements are coming from. A twitch of the wings, and then . . .

Oh crap, someone is talking to me. Time to snap back to attention and act interested in the playgroup conversation. It can be hard to stay tuned in sometimes.

So, when I last touched base with you about my life in Houston, I was talking about expatriate wives and the difficulties I was having with making the type of close friends I'd imagined. My new environment was somewhat strange to me and definitely different from anything I'd experienced before. In my previous life, in engineering and university, I'd become used to guys—men, men, and more men surrounding me, with few other women in the mix. Men had always made up my closest friends and confidantes, and I was used to male interaction.

But here, I was suddenly thrust into this world with all women—privileged women at that—and was supposed to suddenly know how to relate. They weren't like the girls in my Girls' Group. They were, on the whole, more focused on material things and appearances. I didn't know how to talk to them.

Feeling more like an outsider than any real part of the group, I spent a lot of my earlier days just listening to, observing, and analyzing the ladies around me as if they were an odd sociology experiment. The talk was usually light and fluffy. I like to joke about it all being the four C's—children, castle (decorating the house), cooking, and cruising (holiday planning). But more seriously, in light of the depression I was in, I was finding myself bored by it.

How could I care about how much flavor raspberries add to muffins when I was so focused on finding the key to making friends? "What are your deeper thoughts and feelings?" That's what I actually wanted to know. And "how can I connect with you?" (Not that I actually said that, of course!)

Some days, I would feel a bit down and find myself really struggling over the idea that perhaps I was never going to fit in. I mean, what if it was just a fact that no matter what I did, I was never going to click with these ladies as well as they did with each other? What if nobody ever wanted me over or invited me to the more intimate and interesting gatherings? After all, I wasn't one of them.

On those days, the lonely times could become particularly depressing, and they began to feel like a prison sentence that was going to go on and on, and just at a time when I was craving the warmth of company so badly. How I longed to have another house to go to that wasn't my own, that person whom I could drop in on unannounced and always be welcome, any change of scenery other than my own walls, which were starting to feel claustrophobic.

It certainly gave me a new appreciation for my mum's house at home and how comfortable I'd always been dropping by there. I loved how I'd always been free to just spread out on the couch, help myself to food and snacks, and be around someone who was so familiar and welcoming to me. It's amazing what you take for granted and don't notice until it's gone. I guess I was feeling homesick.

Other days, I had a little more spirit and focused on trying to work out my next plan of attack—friendship-wise, that is. Who to approach next and how to approach them. What events or invites could I come up that would interest people?

And while I didn't have a whole lot of success in that, I did learn one thing over the course of my stay with these ladies, and that is that women are complicated. I had no idea how difficult it could be to just communicate "right."

For example, I learnt that if you are a woman yourself, you have to be *really* careful with tone or even avoid saying things in a neutral, direct way, because often, "neutral direct" is how women say unhappy things and "positive fluffy" is how women say okay or good things. It's like a code, and if you get it wrong, others may completely misinterpret your meaning and can take it very badly.

And for the record, I'm not writing these things to complain about women. But I do want to explain how hard it can be for someone who doesn't naturally speak this language to make sense of it. We have to decode it, because this is often a real problem for women Aspies.

At one point, I remember how a friend of mine, Angel, gave me feedback that I said too many things that sounded like complaints, when I really didn't think I did. Her comment really surprised me. But it turned out that many things I'd said were just coming across badly.

For example, saying, "I need help," to somebody who I guess already had been helpful might be taken as, "You're not helping me enough. I'm hinting because I'm disappointed in you." But when I say these things, there's really none of that negativity implied in it. I just mean them as statements of fact. "I'm still so unhappy. I have an issue, and I want you to help me in any way you can." I guess I've never been good at that happy happy, hugs-and-kisses, rainbows-and-kittens language or seeing how others might interpret my words.

A friend of mine, an Aspie mum named Kathy, once told a group of us how her Aspie daughter was learning to speak "Womanese," which I think is a great word for it. It's the language of bending your words to be extremely positive and only presenting your negative comments in flat, neutral hints. It seems that it's a real "must-learn" language for any Aspie girl who doesn't want to be forever frowned upon by other women in her life, although admittedly, it's a skill I'm still a little ordinary at and still improving on myself!

But anyway, enough analysis. I definitely don't want to bore you that way! So it's time for me to move on and tell you some actual stories of the experiences I had.

Over the next however many chapters, I've decided to tell three stories about my experiences with other women in Houston. Two of them, "The Story of Angel" and "The Story of Playgroup B," are examples of troubles I had fitting in socially, where I remain confused about what exactly went wrong. The third, "The Story of Paula," is a happier story to remind us that despite stereotypical behavior, there are always some good people in the world. So let's begin with the more positive one.

CHAPTER FORTY-TWO

THE STORY OF PAULA

I first met Paula at a birthday celebration back in Australia, long before coming to Houston. It was my father-in-law's 60th birthday, and he put on a big show. Paula's husband and my father-in-law were former work colleagues and had kept up with each other as good friends. I remember, at the time of the celebration, Paula was heavily pregnant with her second son and seemed lively and feisty—far too much energy for me! I didn't know her then.

When my husband and I first mentioned going to Houston, my mother-in-law told us the story of her friend Paula who was already over there and suggested we meet up. She told us stories of how Paula had flown over with her second son, only four months old, a similar age to Isaac. She read us letters from Paula and sighed over little unimportant details. She was whimsical about the whole thing.

At first, I groaned at the idea. Most of my mother-in-law's friends are such different personalities from myself. They're all lovely ladies, but in the past, I've found them painfully hard to talk to, so having yet another person with whom I would have to smile and try to uncomfortably get along with sounded like work. But it turned out that in Paula's case, I was wrong.

She was open and compassionate, and I found her easy to open up to. She was capable of intellectual and conceptual thinking as well as the light stuff. In fact, I think Paula is one of those people who has the gift of making anyone feel at ease around her and who fits into conversations with people from all walks of life. I admire her ability to be so versatile. It's certainly not something I could ever do.

After she kindly went out of her way to visit me a few times while settling in, I started taking Isaac to her house to play with her two boys at semi-regular intervals. (We established it was easier for both of us if I came to her.) We had a nice, equal way of interacting, and she was beautifully affectionate with Isaac, who lapped up the attention. She told me about the issues going on in her life, and we connected over missing close friends and family while in Houston.

Paula introduced me to another playgroup of expatriate spouses from her husband's company. (I'll refer to them as Playgroup B for the sake of anonymity.) She made it easy for me to meet them by inviting me to her house one week while she was hosting. Unfortunately, the group did seem a little cliquey, but they were friendly enough about having me off to the side, and it was a great social avenue for Isaac. So I continued to take him along. If nothing else, it got me out of the house! Paula couldn't make most of the meet-ups.

Over our shared time in Houston, Paula got to know me well through our one-on-one chats, and in the end, she turned out to be one of the most supportive friends I had.

As an Aspie, I think it's easy for us to condemn neurotypical people and say they don't care. They're shallow. They're mean to us. It's not worth trying to make typical friends. But every now and then, you come across some non-judgmental, intelligent neurotypicals who can make beautiful comrades. Compassionate people. Deeper, introspective people. People with similar interests to yourself, or those with open minds and beliefs in tolerance. I found several back in Australia, and here was another.

Unfortunately, Paula was also a busy woman, so my time with her was limited. And as her time to leave Houston drew near, she became harder and harder to reach. She was frantic and stressed with organization tasks during the last few months and ended up leaving suddenly when her husband's work finally made a decision on his role. There was no time for farewells, but it was definitely a worthwhile friendship to have had.

I feel especially sad that she's no longer around for Isaac now. He enjoyed her so much. And I still wish she could be around for our boys to grow up together. But unfortunately, that was never a long-term possibility.

Now, going back to discussing my more challenging interactions, it's time for my next Houston expatriate story, the story of Angel.

CHAPTER FORTY-THREE

THE STORY OF ANGEL

It was during one of the weekly expatriate café meetups that I first met Angel. She and another lady, Alexis, were the unofficial leaders of the group and coordinated most of the downtown expatriate events. Angel had sent me an email some months back, shortly after my arrival, to welcome me and let me know that she had a daughter, Isobelle, the same age as my son Isaac. She'd been unable to attend the first month or two of café gatherings I'd come to but commented on how was looking forward to meeting me. It was a very welcoming gesture.

When I first met her in the café, I observed that she was quiet and understated. She appeared formal but simply dressed, with no makeup that stood out to me and long, straight, brown hair parted in the middle. Her face was plain, but overall, she was somehow still quite attractive.

At first, it seemed that perhaps she didn't have a lot to say other than the usual small talk about the weather and simple chit chat; however, as I got to know her, I came to see that she was very much a thinker and analyzer. In fact, she was unusually intelligent in the art of perceiving, understanding, and influencing others.

One day at the weekly lunch, Angel asked me if I wanted to organize some play dates with the kids, so it came about that we began meeting every Thursday afternoon, either at her house or mine. To me, it seemed a reciprocal and positive experience for both the kids and adults involved.

Much later in time—jumping forward for a second—Angel would describe the experience to me as her "reaching out to me to help me" and tell me that the friendship wasn't really enjoyable to her at any point. However, I definitely hadn't picked up any sense of inequality at the time, and I'm usually quick to pick up on those sorts of signals. I study people. So I wonder if it really was because she was that good at acting warm and friendly or if it was hindsight biasing her memories.

I had a few deeper conversations with Angel during this one-on-one time where I expressed my frustrations at how long it was taking me to find "real" friends and settle into a social pattern. It was a hard time in my life, and the issue of isolation had become a focus for me. Angel was most empathetic and pointed out that most of the other ladies had arrived in groups, and I was one of the last to be sent across before the company had decided to limit overseas moves. By the time I arrived, most other expatriates were busy and well settled in. It was bound to be challenging.

She also invited Isaac and me to come join her family for dinner every second Friday when my husband was away at university. Robert, despite my objections, had started an MBA at Tulane, which took him out of the house Friday evenings and most of Saturday and also required extra time for studying and group meetings. My protests that he was away too much had gone unheard, so now I was struggling to cope with not five but six twelve-hour days alone.

The dinners broke up the long, most difficult days, and watching Isaac play with Isobelle and Angel's husband, Hayden, made me smile. With so little family and friends around, I was so relieved for Isaac to have other regular adults in his life, and I really valued this time.

Hayden was fantastic with the children and especially entertaining to watch as he invented games that made them giggle and squeal. They emptied Angel's Tupperware out of her cupboards and made great wet messes with the little splash trough she had outside on her deck. Hayden was a fantastic cook and baked homemade gourmet pizzas and other tasty meals to share with us.

Things seemed to be going well for me on that level, at least. Then one day, I made a brave decision to talk to Angel about Asperger's Syndrome . . . and that's when something went wrong. I'll never be sure exactly what, but something did, and it was *very* wrong.

My decision to talk to Angel about Asperger's came after many months of researching the condition and keeping it to myself. At first, I hadn't told anyone but my husband about this idea I had, because after all, how do you bring up such a personal topic to somebody you're only just getting to know when you're not even sure yourself what's going on? Angel was the only local person I spoke to regularly (Paula wasn't regularly in the picture yet), so there wasn't anyone else for me to open up to.

However, in late September 2010, when I went to the first of my two official diagnostic sessions, I was left just buzzing with things to say. So many unexplained troubles in my life had been suddenly and so simply explained in the course of just a few hours talking to a counselor. I no longer had any doubt that I had Asperger's. I couldn't believe the revelations I'd had.

I decided that Angel was a person I trusted enough to share this incredible discovery with. With my mind racing with a combination of relief, sadness, and a hint of annoyance for everything I'd gone through unnecessarily, I wrote to her to organize a meetup.

In my buzz, I also wrote a post on Facebook saying I needed a friendly ear. My friend Carina from the hotel asked me if I wanted to drive up and see her, so I jumped on the invitation and went up to her house the next day. So in the end, I found two people to talk with. I'll discuss how things went with Carina a bit later in the book, but her response was pretty straightforward.

With Angel, however, things suddenly became confusing. I made a time to come see her at her house the day after I met up with Carina, and I had a long chat with her about Asperger's and what it meant for me. I went into detail on some little things that have been challenging for me, my past, my difficulties with the current group settings, and how I'd been lonely here.

As with Carina, I was doing most of the talking that day, but it seemed to go down okay. I told her all about the diagnostic process and how I was looking forward to hearing the results. And admittedly, I probably did get a bit teary that day as I was confiding in her about some of my past hardships and might have Aspie'd her with a few too many depressing details.

After all, after just finding out about my AS, it was hard not to feel a degree of self-pity over the various ways I'd had to suffer unnecessarily in life, at least temporarily. So once I started on the topic, I was so relieved to just tell someone, I couldn't stop talking. I know I could hear myself going on and on, but it was like releasing the valve on the bottom of a water tank. It just had to come out! But Angel was patient with me, and it made me feel a lot better. I walked away feeling positive about giving her an update next week.

The next week, Angel rang me and asked if I minded her adding a few additional ladies to our playgroup that Thursday. I agreed it was fine, as I thought I could benefit from making one or two more friends in a more intimate environment. It would be an initial effort, but I assessed it to be worth the cost. I thought perhaps she was even trying to help me get to know some of the other ladies in this smaller setting. Then, suddenly, the group was very large. It was a little more than I'd expected.

Angel also mentioned to me that she was having trouble accommodating all the ladies on the Thursday and wanted to move the day of the week. I replied that that was fine with me so long as it wasn't a Tuesday. Tuesday mornings, I had my Playgroup B mums' group, the only other thing on my schedule, and with Isaac's sleep patterns as they were, I couldn't realistically attend both. Not to mention how exhausting that would be for me!

Within two weeks of our initial discussion, the playgroup had been moved to a Tuesday, and I was told, "Sorry, but I can't please everybody, and I had to make a decision," and that my reasons were less compelling than the other ladies'. As a founder of the group, I was disappointed and felt it was rather inconsiderate toward me. But as I knew these ladies better than the Playgroup B people, I decided to drop my group B and come along anyway. Angel reassured me that it was nothing to do with me, and "as a leader, sometimes you have to make tough calls."

After that, there seemed to be a lot of other little things happening that made it difficult for me to attend, but always for a good reason. I mentioned to Angel once that (now pregnant with Trent) I was having an issue with making it to the furthest parks without a bathroom. My bladder wasn't holding up to the drive back. By coincidence, the group that week was permanently moved to the park furthest from me, one that happened not to have a bathroom.

Of course, it was because it had a splash area and the kids were enjoying the water in the heat of summer, and I did hear comments from some of the other ladies on how much they liked that park.

One week, construction work was going on, and a port-a-loo was put up temporarily. I told Angel I was looking forward to coming along, as I hadn't been in a while. That week, she sent out an email to the group suggesting we could either go to the park or better, to a friend Tiffany's pool instead, and requested people ring Tiffany if they planned to go.

I didn't usually attend the pool gatherings nor did I like ringing people (as Angel knew), but I was so keen to see people, I rang Tiffany and arranged to come anyway. The email had implied that the pool was the option of choice. Later in the day, Tiffany rang me back to ask if I wanted to cancel, as I was the only one who'd replied. It turned out Angel had contacted the regulars privately and organized for them to meet at the park after all. I guess she didn't include me.

Previously, Angel and I had spent the odd Wednesday morning at the Children's Museum of Houston together with the kids. From that Wednesday onward, she invited along another lady, Ebony, and they talked closely while I seemed to be always off to the side.

Now, it's most likely that my separation here was due to my difficulties joining in on a three-way conversation in the loud setting with the distraction of kids than any sort of specific exclusion, but it all added up to one pattern. Angel was never alone with me again (barring the two catch ups discussed below) and never had to "talk" to me about anything personal again.

One day, for no apparent reason, she sent me the details of a few other mums' groups in the area she thought I might "like to join" (instead). I hadn't indicated that I wished to join anywhere else.

Now, am I imagining all this, or was I being pushed out? Certainly, each thing that happened (and many other little such things) wasn't, on its own, something I would think too much of. Some of them, I'm sure, didn't mean anything. But all put together, it was adding up to something odd, and it would seem that at the least she was certainly being inconsiderate of me—me, who she knew was challenged already and was going to be strongly affected by her actions. It did seem a rather unfriendly thing to do.

But all the while, Angel was positive and warm in person and assured me that we were good friends. It made me so confused, and I found myself questioning my ability to even read the situation.

While I still had faith in her, I tried reaching out via email and explaining to her that I still wanted one-on-one time occasionally. I sent her a short paragraph written by Tony Attwood explaining why it's hard for an Aspie to follow a larger group conversation. I thought it would help her understand. But she didn't seem interested and explained she was unable to accommodate me. She was "too busy" by then.

When we did catch a moment, she gave me a lot of advice on things I should say or do with other people to make friends while keeping me at arm's length herself. Eventually, I did manage to corner her to have a proper talk about what was going on. The feeling of separation had been bothering me, and I needed to resolve it by talking things through.

At first, Angel repeated that everything was good and that we were friends. But when I pressed her about one-on-one time, she eventually confessed that she didn't like talking to me alone. She said I talked too much about myself and was frustrating to try and "help." She explained that I didn't ask other people enough questions to follow up on their lives or put enough effort into the friendship and so on, with various other reasons why I wasn't that fun to be friends with.

Of course, it was said in a kind, positive context, as if she were the good guy helping me with constructive criticism. I'm sure my paraphrasing of it sounds far, far more negative than the way it was conveyed, but I guess that's how I heard it. And then that was the last one-on-one gathering I ever managed to make with her.

I guess I'll never know if it was the knowledge of my Asperger's Syndrome that put her off or just my lack of gratitude and failure to respond to her attempts to "fix" me. She said her driver was wanting to help people, though I imagine having others who think you're a wonderful, selfless, and altruistic person whom they are indebted to could be the more appealing part. I wasn't changing in response to her advice or acting grateful but instead was resisting and trying to explain why the changes didn't and couldn't work for me. She didn't want to hear those explanations.

I'm also perhaps not the sort of person who is good at showing gratitude in the conventional happy, flowery ways. I suppose this does look unappreciative to someone who doesn't understand me well.

Anyway, after our chat, some of her words really sank in and started to get me down, because the things she pointed out were mostly my Aspie tendencies. It got into my head and made me start doubting my worth as a person. I couldn't completely help the faults she was highlighting. After all, they're part of what being an Aspie embodies. But in her eyes, such traits were deal breakers, and no one could ever be friends with such a person. Would I never really be likable to anybody as myself? She certainly seemed to think not.

I suddenly needed to get out of there and went on an impromptu holiday to Australia to see my old friends. It was rushed, I know, but with me so depressed at home, I suggested it, and Robert just made it happen. I don't think I even said goodbye to many of the ladies in Houston or told them I was leaving. It was a quick decision, and I was down and not in the mood to act happy or bring it up with people. And thank heavens I went home. It made a lot of difference.

Being back in Australia reminded me that there are many people who value me for who I am, differences and all. I was reassured that, thankfully, Angel's view wasn't shared by everyone. Angel was seeing her vision of who she thought I should be and the deficit between that and who I was. But she wasn't seeing the good in who I was. She's never seen my cheeky humor or how I engage with others when I'm happy. She doesn't know what a loyal and compassionate friend I can be. She just saw that I didn't fit into the mold of what she looks for in a person and completely failed to value the rest.

When I came back, Angel seemed to have "forgotten" completely about the Friday dinners or making any contact with me at all, and she never did ask me anything about my Asperger's or the results of my diagnosis. I guess for all the talk of being friends, she wasn't really interested in hearing about me. But she remained exceptionally friendly and enthusiastic in her chats to me whenever I saw her in the group. Any onlooker would have thought we were best buddies!

Chapter Forty-Four

Misunderstanding and Causing Offense

Q: You've talked about being rejected and about the sudden loss of friends
before. Do you think there could be a pattern to the way this comes about?

Unfortunately, yes. I'm concerned that there might be.

While this may have been the most extreme case, I've had a few instances where
someone I thought I was close to suddenly seemed annoyed and distant with me and I
never knew why. And it has hurt and perplexed me every time.

I've deliberated a lot over the years about that handful of people I've lost or annoyed in my life and realized that I think causing offense to others without intending
to do so must just come as part of Aspie territory. Perhaps I say or do things every now
and then that people find distasteful. I have enough evidence to indicate that I must.

But it can be hard to know what and when, because people rarely react straight
away, and sometimes they don't ever admit it directly. To me, it is more likely to come
across as someone suddenly going off me for reasons unknown. One minute, everything seems good, and then the next, I sense coolness and hostility, as if I'm supposed
to be aware of the crime I've committed. Of course, it's usually a mystery to me!

I believe part of the problem is that often, the "crime" committed is only others'
misinterpretation of something I've done or said (or an expression I made), when, in
fact, there was no mal intent at all. For example, I've heard descriptions of how when

Aspies tune out or look away, we can appear aloof or disinterested in the conversation, when in reality, we may just be preoccupied with a random thought or idea.

People will take offense to the things they perceive because they assume it means the same thing that it would mean if *they* looked away or made that expression. We're "dismissing" them. They don't check with us to learn why we did it or what we really intended by it, which is a big problem when you consider that Aspie and typical communication and expressions are worlds apart!

I remember one of the expatriate mums, Samina, explaining to me much later in time that I'd offended Angel by "throwing the friendship in her face" and that's why she acted as she did. At the time of the conversation, I nodded and agreed, yet when I thought about it later, I had no idea what I'd done that would have constituted that. I nodded because I just assumed she must be right. I must have caused offense, because that's "what I do," and I never did get a chance to ask for further clarification.

Looking back, I still don't know what that actually means. I know once Angel told me she didn't want me as a one-on-one friend anymore, I became guarded and was no longer as open as I used to be. But I remained polite to her out and about. I'm not aware of anything else negative that I'm guilty of.

I guess the most likely explanation is that perhaps Angel interpreted me badly on occasion and wasn't the sort of person who asked for clarification. I'm not sure in regard to what, but for most people, I know perception of subtle things is what they go by, and if you appear to be doing something negative, then apparently that's what you're doing.

It takes time for people to really get to know us and how we tick before they figure out how to take us. Did I frown the wrong way? I have no awareness of my facial expression. Did I fail to open up and talk and question the way I was supposed to? I'll probably never know. But I know I wasn't feeling mean or aggressive at heart, just hurt and afraid to trust her again for a while there, I guess.

It's all a moot point now. That friendship is long gone, and I haven't seen Angel now for some years, but I wonder if that all could have turned out differently had she ever asked me what I meant by things instead of just taking it whatever way she did.

As my high school friend Emma once put it, "If Michelle said it, just assume it wasn't meant as badly as it sounded."

CHAPTER FORTY-FIVE

DIFFICULTY SNAPPING IN AND OUT OF TASKS

Now, here is a topic for any of you readers who have had the, um . . . "pleasure" of living with one of us Aspies, which I'm going to go ahead and define as a good thing overall. It's good, right, so no saying otherwise!

But as good as I'm saying we are, I know that one of the areas we can be a tiny bit difficult in (okay, okay, one of many) is that we do tend to be a little, um, not the best when interrupted in the middle of focusing hard on our task at hand. It's a bit of an Aspie thing.

In fact, as mentioned earlier, in an online study on Aspie behaviors where over two hundred thousand people were questioned, one of the questions with the highest number of "yes" responses from Aspies was, "Does it feel vitally important to be left undisturbed when focusing on your special interests?"[47] with the questions, "Do you become frustrated if an activity that is important to you gets interrupted?" and, "Do you tend to get so absorbed by your special interests that you forget or ignore everything else?" also ranking very highly.

So it really is a predominant Aspie trait. Hyperfocus, which I value highly, can make us wonderful achievers in our areas of interest, but unfortunately, it also comes with a downside in that it can make us easily agitated to the point of meltdown. It's

---

[47] "Aspie-Quiz evaluation," RDOS website, as at 08/05/2012, http://www.rdos.net/eng/aspeval/

why many Aspies lose jobs and act up at work. Social and sensory overstimulation, combined with frequent interruptions, builds our stress levels to the point where we can't handle it anymore. We're not wired for all this chopping and changing that typical people like to do.

I know for me, when I'm working hard, even the slightest interruptions are incredibly grating. They require me to let go of what I'm doing and (slowly) alter my mind to pay attention to the social world again. In the process of "mental shifting" before I've fully disengaged, there is always an interim point where I'm agitated but haven't yet fully moved back into social awareness. I may not register the person interrupting me as a person for a few seconds, and I can be susceptible to barking at them for the interruption.

It's a situation that I am careful not to put myself in nowadays, because I don't want to treat the people I love that way. However, growing up, I'm afraid this is something most of my family witnessed!

For someone who doesn't understand, it's easy to mistake an Aspie's apparent annoyance at being interrupted as merely bad temper. However, we're not getting agitated for no reason. Our brain wiring means that these interruptions really do cause us tremendous stress at the time, so it's not a case of us just not *wanting* to switch back and forth between our work and the person talking to us. We're genuinely not able to do this as rapidly or as easily as neurotypical people.

So, what is there to do about it? Heaven knows. I have absolutely no idea! I guess it's just always going to take a little patience from both sides.

CHAPTER FORTY-SIX

THE STORY OF PLAYGROUP B

Now, wandering onto my next story of social struggles. Fun, fun . . .

After returning from Australia, I gave up on trying to attend Angel's playgroups. I was starting to suffer from a pregnancy complication (pelvic instability) that made it painful for me to walk around, and chasing Isaac about the park was way beyond my abilities.

For some reason, the expatriate weekly café meetups had also ceased by the time I got back. Odd. But I began attending Playgroup B again and took consolation that at least Isaac was getting some socialization from that! Luckily, the Playgroup B gatherings were all in people's houses, and I could sit without having to worry about Isaac running away—and believe me, when you're the sore mother of an energetic two-year-old, that's a big plus!

When I returned to Playgroup B, it surprised me to see how much it had changed from the good ol' days when I used to attend. The members had almost completely turned over, and I wondered where so many of the former ladies had gone. I guess many had returned home or perhaps just stopped attending. I couldn't say. Either way, I was happy to see so many friendly and lively new characters and sense such a positive, welcoming air to the new group.

Being able to attend the group, of course, did come with the drawback of having to host the group myself every month or two—grumble grumble—which could feel like a slow form of Aspie torture. I wish it was polite to put signs all over my stuff saying "don't touch," "only sit in these areas," and "no crumbs" and then kick everybody out the second I felt I'd had enough. But alas, that doesn't go down so well in the NT world!

So I managed to endure it for the sake of pulling my weight. And overall, with so many ladies new to the area, I felt in a good position to connect with those who wanted to get to know people and could use help and company upon settling in. It gave me hope that finally I could make some stable friends!

So what went wrong this time? Well, that's a tough question, one I'm still stumped by. All I can say is perhaps we could call it a clash of personality. Or could it have been another Aspie-not-knowing-how-to-communicate-with-somebody moment or simply a person just not being nice to me? I'm unsure, so I'll let you decide. Here's what happened:

Come the last trimester of my pregnancy, I began to feel increasingly sore from moving about and even bending to clean or picking toys up, so I decided that hosting the group was going to be off the table for a while. I needed as little on my plate as possible to allow me to rest and recover, so when the next roster came out, I wrote my apologies to the organizer, Becky, explaining the mobility difficulties I was having and how I wanted a break from hosting this round.

Becky replied to me quickly, saying that it wasn't a problem and giving me a few words of best wishes for the pregnancy. And that was it. I was pleasantly surprised it was so easy, and I thanked her for her understanding. She wasn't the sort of person I'd expected empathy from, and it was a big relief. It seemed like it had been sorted out and all was well.

A week or two later when the next round of playgroups commenced, however, I noticed that I hadn't been forwarded the address details for the next group. Puzzled, I sent an email to my friend Paula to check if the playgroup was on, and she got back to me verifying it. She also told me that she'd talked to Becky to ask her to include me, and Becky told her that I'd opted out of the playgroup.

That perplexed me, as I was pretty sure I'd been clear in my request. But regardless, I wrote back to Becky explaining there was a misunderstanding and how I really did want to come to the playgroups. I explained again that it was just the hosting that I wasn't up to. After all, these groups were the only time I could get Isaac around other children, and I was already feeling terribly guilty for not being able to socialize and exercise him enough.

That was when I found out I'd apparently done something wrong. The reply I got took me aback. Becky informed me, somewhat bluntly, that it's the policy of the group that everyone must host in order to be able to attend. She apologized and wrote that "other ladies have had babies, and they managed to host," and that I could rejoin the group once I had specified a date that I was going to host. "We all pull our weight. Sorry." For now, I was out.

Now, please tell me I'm not crazy in thinking that was a cold way to dismiss someone. After all, the key function of this group was supposed to be a social support network, but when I genuinely found myself in a time of need, the group wasn't flexible enough to include me. It didn't seem cool.

I suppose I could've just agreed and picked a date just after Trent's birth to comply or called Becky to talk about the situation (eugh, phone calls!), but something in me had a strong gut resistance to the way I'd been pressured to host. It seemed almost, to exaggerate, a little like bullying. So, stunned and somewhat stubborn, I didn't reply immediately.

After that, I never did hear from any of the ladies in the group again, which was sad, as I think various individuals in the group could've been nice. My decision not to chase it up came after the next meetup, when I heard through a friend how Becky had had a bit of a bitch about me to the group that week, the basis being, "If she can go to groups, then she can host them," and complaining about me trying to get out of contributing. Even my friend said at the time that she couldn't really argue with that.

It definitely put me off thinking of the group as kind and supportive or wanting to be there again. I didn't like the idea of having to debate and play politics just to push myself back in after I'd been shown so little consideration, or facing the "bad reputation" that I might now have. So I guess that's the story of how I became at odds with Playgroup B.

I can reflect now and see that had I been someone else or in a more positive state, I could have perhaps tried to contact some of the other ladies and organize my own social gatherings. There are other ways I could have pursued friendship. But I guess at the time, I was feeling a little too down to have the energy to keep trying. It's one of those unfortunate things that depression can do to you. I started to give up and let my self-talk convince me that I just wasn't wanted by the other people. I guess I'll never know what the other ladies actually thought of it all.

After that hiccup, I found myself at a most isolated and solitary period in my life. I had about a month where I didn't see a single other person I knew except for my husband, and that was for brief periods. All the while, I struggled to keep up with Isaac for the long days alone and was badly in need of help. It was one of my most depressing times, and I can understand completely why solitary confinement is torture. Something in your head just wants to scream, "End this! End this now!" But somehow, although it felt like years, I did get through it, minute by minute, hour by hour, day by day.

Going through this experience certainly did get me thinking about a lot of things. One question that kept coming to me was why am I so bad at finding help when I need it? I presume this has something to do with not knowing how to ask for it to endear people to want to help. I suppose most people maintain a level of constant communication with each other that compels them to want to be involved as troubles arise. However, in my new country, I hadn't yet found such a sounding board.

At the time, I made hints on Facebook that I was in want of company, but they seemed to mostly go ignored. I wrote a letter one day just to get all the words out, but it was mostly just an exercise in venting. I had no audience for it. (You can read the letter below.)

I noticed a pattern—whenever I attempted to ask for help, others didn't seem to take me seriously. I wondered if people heard me and thought, "Well, you have all these people around you. You have no cause for complaint. If you're not getting along with others, it's because of your own aloof/[insert other word here] attitude," or, "You're just looking for pity or attention."

Is it that people just don't believe the magnitude of what I'm expressing? Or they do and they dismiss it? I wonder why.

Come the end of my pregnancy, Trent arrived with no baby shower or local friends anticipating his arrival. We had no visitors at the hospital, and I was so conscious of how far this was from my dreams of bringing him into a world with a loving community around to welcome and celebrate him. I felt like I let him down as a mother. I'd wanted to be able to give him so much more.

Fortunately, his life and social circles have picked up a lot since then, and he never suffered in any way. But I remember that, at the time, it was heartbreaking for me.

My email to an imaginary person:

> I am writing this email because I need to reach out to someone and say, "Help." I'm really not okay. I keep falling into a sort of isolation and depression that I just can't seem to snap myself out of.
>
> I know when I was pregnant with my first son, Isaac, I did get a little emotional and down at this early stage, so I'm sure hormones are compounding it. But this time, it's worse, because I'm so alone through it. I've felt isolated for a while now, and I'm starting to realize that this isn't just a transition period. I'm simply not making friends here, and perhaps I'm not the sort of person who can.
>
> Before you object, I realize I do have lots of people around me. People who I see at playgroups and our own mothers group. People who I seem to get along well with and who are nice to me.

However, I'm not really becoming close to any one of them. I think the problem may be that the way I connect with real friends is so different from what these groups are offering. I'm not good at small talk. In the group settings, I can't follow the conversation and relax and be the real me. I'm not making personal connections this way. I walk away unsatisfied, feeling like I haven't really opened my heart to anyone.

I value real, deep, one-on-one conversation with people I can talk to privately and be myself around. Yet, having said that, if you do catch me one-on-one, I can't even guarantee I'll talk. I take a while to get over being self-conscious with people I don't know well. I fear the awkward silences. So you see, it's hopeless. I want close, deep, and meaningful friendships, and I'm never going to start one with people whom I only see twice a week in a big crowd.

I've been in Houston a year now, and I think this is where I'm getting so lost:

- I'm not the sort of person who knows how to initiate a conversation with someone.

- I don't know how to ask for help when I need it, especially when I need it badly.

- I don't know how to initiate outings or call upon someone when I'm alone and really need company that day.

- I don't know how to find out what people are doing and when and how to get myself invited to these things.

- I feel very uncomfortable calling people on the phone. If I don't have something specific I want, then what's my opening line? It's too stressful for me.

- I don't even know if I can be the sort of friend the conventional way that people seem to want.

- Heck, I'm not good at communication in general.

I don't really know what I want from you in writing this. I suppose it's to let someone know that I am socially stuck and I need someone to be here with me, just someone to be around and to talk to when I really need to talk, because I don't know how I'm going to make it through the rest of this week with my husband away for large "As it stands, the legislation is thinly disguised anti-gay Christian bigotry, pure and simple. The bill is a naked attempt to force Christian theocracy upon the citizens of Oklahoma."the next day or even the next hour. I spend over seventy hours a week completely alone, bar my son and the other strangers I see in the street.

I'm so unhappy here. I miss home, and I just need to put that out there and reach out to somebody—ANYBODY—rather than sit home and self-destruct!

Michelle

CHAPTER FORTY-SEVEN

ACTING THE NT PART AND FEELING "FAKE"

I was having a discussion with a fellow Aspie, David N., the other day about how sometimes in social settings, we can get the feeling that we're being "fake." He told me how he's always felt like a fraud, as if he's acting and being someone who isn't himself, because he knows deep down that the real him doesn't belong. Both of us agreed that we (and probably many other Aspies) find this feeling uncomfortable because we don't like dishonesty and pretense. To my friend, it was just another thing he detested about himself. He said he never understood where that feeling was coming from.

In my mind, it's been clear to me for a while why I feel that way. It's because, to fit in properly, as Aspies, we're often "acting" the neurotypical role. To fully integrate, society demands that we adjust our behavior strongly so that we no longer feel genuine about who we are. Some of us fall so deeply into this role, we lose ourselves and forget the things that make us unique—our uniqueness, our humor, the activities that give us joy. Many of us do learn to play this role and even play it well. Some have more trouble with it. A few don't even try. But the real question is, should we?

Since I've (recently) stopped trying to be like everyone else and pass as a neurotypical quite as much, I've found myself so much happier in life. More authentic. While some people in my life may shun the Aspie traits I display, many also love them. It surprises me how many people find the quirks charming and amusingly typical. Suppressing them, it turns out, isn't always the best answer, and it certainly isn't a satisfying one.

So I guess the key is in finding a balance—changing the big and easy-to-change issues that cause the most offense but not changing so much that it becomes constant work or you start not to feel like yourself. I think owning your inner Aspie, combined with confidence in who you are, leads to the most satisfying, successful sort of life.

One thing that always concerns me is when I hear people or organizations talking about "training" young Aspies to live a more normal life. I agree that learning and knowing the skills could be helpful, but what I don't like about it is the subtle pressure that it could put on Aspies to change and become the neurotypical way completely. There's an unavoidable underlying message: Who you are isn't right, and this is what you should be instead.

I want to tell those young Aspies and their parents that while skills and knowing social norms is great, never forget to value yourself (or your child) for who you are and all the great things that make up you. To parents, encourage some of the fun quirks. Let them flap around if they want to. Who is it hurting anyway? Teens are particularly impressionable about not seeing the good in themselves and having a hard time with being different. Aspie teens need the adults in their lives to show it to them.

Similarly, when I hear about workplace initiatives to train Aspies and help them find jobs, I wonder is it a complete service that includes making sure they are truly okay in the workplace in the long term, or does it just stop at how to "do everything right"? An Aspie can learn to do a job well, but acting in "the right way" over long periods of time takes its toll. We Aspies need to be okay in a more sustainable way.

Look at someone like myself, for example. I never got fired. I did my jobs well, sometimes exceptionally. But I was far from okay doing it. The focus in my working life had always been about me doing whatever it took to fit into the role and never on what I needed to be contented in the job. It's like the cliché of the round peg in a square hole. I can learn easily enough to bend that way, but over time, it gets uncomfortable. I start to suffer for it. Instead of continually trying to squash myself into that square, what I need is for the workplace to cut me a rounder hole.

Give me some space and some time to do things in my own way. Let me come and go as I need to get the work done, and stop expecting me to always be doing so much of those little social/political things that exhaust me so. There are a million other employees who could do those things instead. I never did understand why it was so critical that every employee do their own calling around and schmoozing.

It just makes sense to re-delegate it, because while stifled, an Aspie may still work okay, but half their energy is wasted on just coping with being there. In comparison, a comfortable, focused Aspie can do amazing things. Let us work our magic the way we do best.

There's so much joy in being free to really do what you do well and have other people appreciate you for your authentic self. I want every Aspie to know that feeling.

Chapter Forty-Eight

Life in Houston— Expatriate Mums, Part Two

And so my story continues:

A few weeks before my son Trent was born, my mum flew in from Australia to help out. It was a great relief for me. Having someone to play with Isaac, finally having some company after such a difficult period, and having a person to talk to again made such a world of difference. Feeling better for the first time in some months, I picked up quickly and got on with enjoying baby preparations, although in the back of my mind, I did have a niggling fear about how life might fall back into that lonely place after she left.

It was in this time I also started to go to regular Aspie meetups and really connect with other Aspies. I made some new friends. We formed the League that I talked about earlier, and I found myself suddenly inspired and busy with new and exciting things. And I'm happy to report that my fears were unwarranted, and I didn't ever find myself quite that lonely again—quite the opposite, in fact. My social life was about to expand from then on.

On the downside, it was around six months after Trent was born that Robert and I separated, though in an amicable way. Robert had dreams of traveling around the world to pursue his career, whereas I insisted on settling in one place and really wanted somebody to be around and give a lot more attention to me and the boys. But I have to say, Robert has been very generous about supporting and setting up me and the kids after the separation. He could have walked away and left me—an Aspie mum with two young kids—to try and cope on my own, but he didn't.

He set us up in a nice house and helped me sort out all the paperwork and moving complications. He remained available and is still always just a phone call away to help out if I'm having trouble sorting out paperwork or don't know how to handle something. He also calls most days to just sit and listen to the boys play in the evening and talk to them if they want to chat. He's positive and encourages them to treat Mummy well, keeping in mind that the happier I am, the better all our lives will be, and he visits when he can. I've been very, *very* lucky to have someone so mature and reasonable to co-parent with.

So that all sounds a bit sad, but in the long run, things did work themselves out toward a happier ending, and I guess I learnt a few things about myself along the way. I've learnt that I'm not made for being uprooted and thrown into new social adventures. Some expatriate ladies love the experience (and compensation) of moving country every two to four years, and in theory, it does sound stimulating. But in practice, I need time to develop new friendships and seek out the people who are right for me. In two years, I'm really only just getting started. I'd already ruled out a life of upheaval for the sake of the children, but now I'm certain of it for my sake as well.

I've also learnt that trying to socialize with whoever is thrown in my path isn't necessarily the best approach for me. The people who are right for me are those rare ones who enrich my life and encourage me to be myself and follow the dreams that inspire me. They're hard to come by, but the alternative of trying to win the approval of people with closed minds and set views on behavior deflates me and can only leave me unsatisfied.

And I see that taking such friendships to heart and doing whatever it takes to repair them can be damaging to my own self-worth. So perhaps it means that in the future, I'll walk away from some people more quickly. But it'll be worth it to surround myself with that 5 percent with whom I can really be myself and shine. I deserve to be happy too.

CHAPTER FORTY-NINE

TELLING YOUR CHILD THEY HAVE ASPERGER'S

Q: I'd like some advice. I have a child/teen with Asperger's Syndrome. Do you think I should tell them about it?

Yes, absolutely.

As an adult who was diagnosed late, I often lament how much easier my life could have been had I only known about my Asperger's Syndrome earlier and had time to get a good grasp on myself and my needs.

I think back to my first job and how I would probably have been allowed part-time work had I been able to justify my reasons for wanting it or the various other workplace changes that I could have asked for if anyone had ever pinpointed to me exactly where my difficulties lay. At the time, I found it so hard to put my finger on where this frustration was coming from. I sought answers but took years to figure it out by myself. I needed someone to spell it out.

"The cubicle environment is too bright and noisy. Having people wandering around and interacting with me when I'm trying to focus irritates and exhausts me. Networking and communication tasks aren't a good fit for me." And so on. And to think, all along, there was published material out there that could have helped!

I also think about how much of my life I've spent *forcing* myself to do things that were *really not okay* for me because they were the standard expectations of other people, going to functions or celebrations and trying to mingle for the duration because I was expected to be there (and it would be impolite to leave), doing workplace tasks such as calling around to chase up work, and networking with suppliers to "keep on top of new innovations."

These jobs, to most people, aren't a big deal, but for me, they require so much will-power to get into the high-energy concentrate-and-say-the-right-thing mode required. And having to do them in the daily work environment evoked a certain dread. But I was so afraid back then that people would think I was lazy or apathetic if I avoided work, so I kept beating myself up and pushing through it.

Imagine how that would have changed if I'd known about my Asperger's then. In-stead of questioning and criticizing myself, I could have been looking for solutions and explaining my needs to others. Maybe the people around me would have been okay with me avoiding some of the people-oriented jobs. Maybe I could have felt justified in changing tasks around a little or even saying no some of the time!

It could have made all the difference between me being okay and not okay. Per-haps my career could have turned out differently. I can be incredibly industrious when functioning at optimum levels. But instead, I was forever running on low, battling ex-haustion, frustration, and a general urge to get out of there. What a waste of my talents.

Knowing there's a real reason for my difficulties makes a lot of difference.

And going even deeper again, imagine going through life repeatedly at odds with people and never understanding where others' negative reactions are coming from. Imagine all the horrible assumptions you might make about yourself in response to that.

I think most people with Asperger's will experience other people reacting badly to something they did or said at least every now and then. And if you know that you have Asperger's, you can dismiss it as Aspie behavior and misunderstanding. But when you spend a large part of your life having these experiences and never knowing why, it's only natural to start to wonder what's wrong with you. You begin to look for pat-terns and make assumptions such as, "There's something wrong/bad/boring/negative underneath, and when people get to know me, they'll see it and walk away."

I remember a point in my life where I came up with a theory based on how fre-quently my friendships petered out. "It must be because after a while, people get sick of me and don't want to spend time with me anymore. After all, I do tend to go on about things. I must just be an unlikeable person." That was what my inner voice was telling me.

Just recently, a friend in my Aspie group, David N., was telling a story about a recurring dream that he has. It was something along the lines of being at a campfire or social gathering where people are laughing and socializing in a group, and he stands there in the background, a demented, grotesque figure hiding in the bushes. He wants to join in, but he's afraid that if he comes out into the light, the others will see what a hideous creature he is, so he holds back.

This is a picture analogy for how he feels in life. He has explained before how he had formed an inner belief that there must be something wrong, bad, or ugly within, and when people get to know him, they start to see it and turn away.

This man is the most humble, considerate, kind, and nurturing person I've ever met. There is nothing ugly about him inside or out. He shows wisdom, intelligence, and a great deal of understanding toward those around him. He goes out of his way to be supportive and encouraging. I couldn't think of anything further from the truth than his ugly vision of himself. But fifty-plus years of negative vibes from other people have cemented this idea in his head, and once such ideas are in your head, they're hard to get out.

Sometimes I think of myself as part of a lost generation (or generations), the ones who had to go through life with Asperger's unknowingly. And I'm hoping that in the future, with better education and understanding, the Aspie youth of the future will have a completely different experience.

I've read quite a few postings online from people who were diagnosed late, expressing how indignant and irritated they are that all the time, this was what they had and they never knew it. They felt irritated that the world never cut them a break and about all the instances in their life where, had others been understanding, things could have been so much easier. They're perturbed by all the internal anxiety they'd put themselves through unnecessarily.

It's a nice feeling—a relief—to finally find an explanation for all the confusion and difficulties in your life, but it would have been even nicer to have known it all along.

In a schooling situation, I think revealing one's Asperger's becomes more complex. Do you tell the teachers about it? Probably, provided they are good teachers. Is it beneficial to tell the other students? I'm not sure. I haven't experienced being labeled with Asperger's in a high school situation, so I don't know if having the label and standing out would be more problematic than the symptoms themselves. Teenagers can be very cruel in taunting those who are different. If the teachers led by positive example and encouraged the right sort of attitude, I think it could work out well. But attitudes vary.

I don't have the answers, but I do think that regardless of what you decide about the teachers and other students, it's important to let the child know about their own Asperger's. It enables them to understand themselves better and form the right sort of self-beliefs and attitude.

So my opinion is, *do* tell your children they have Asperger's. Tell them in age-appropriate, positive ways. Let them know they have a special mind and that it comes with blessings as well. Because I think nobody should have to go through life with this syndrome not knowing what it is.

CHAPTER FIFTY

TELLING OTHERS ABOUT MY ASPERGER'S

Q: So, why don't you tell people about your Asperger's Syndrome then?

Ah, that is a perceptive question. What a smart imaginary question-asker I have here!

Since I wrote the early chapters of this book, things have changed a lot for me, and I think you'll see that my mindset on how to approach my Asperger's has also been slowly shifting. I'm starting to see that hiding it from others may not actually be such a good thing. In fact, the more I learn about it, the more confidence I have about it. And I find myself suddenly no longer afraid of people leaving me if I reveal my Asperger's to them.

It's an empowering feeling, actually, to let go of that fear and be open with people about who I am, and in the future, I'd like to head more and more in that direction. But learning about my Asperger's self has been a journey, and it took me quite a while to even get to this point.

Back when I first began to really understand what Asperger's Syndrome is, I was living in a new country with few people I knew well. In fact, it was this isolation and dfficulty finding my feet that drove me to dig into it in the first place. At first, this Asperger's discovery of mine was just a theory, a thought of, "You know what? I really do have a few of these traits."

And then I started reading online accounts of what having Asperger's really feels like to other Aspies, and all of a sudden, it hit me. I wasn't just a little bit Aspie. This was me. Everything these people were saying—the stories being related—were completely me, and it was the most amazing discovery. Painted with an Aspie brush, for the first time, my life began to make sense.

Once I got a taste of Asperger's knowledge, I wanted to learn everything there was to know about it, and I wanted to tell the world. I was excited, thinking finally I was going to have a way to explain myself to people, and they would accept me better. And so I chose to tell two of my close friends, Carina and Angel, about my new discovery (as I described before). I was looking forward to it bringing us closer and being a bonding experience for everyone. But for some reason, both times, it didn't go down too well.

Carina seemed okay while I was talking to her and was supportive and non-judgmental. We talked about me coming up to her house for regular weekly visits to have a stable social activity. She was enthusiastic and actually told me it made sense and it was all cool. But over the course of the day, I think I may have been guilty of Aspie-ing her with a crazy amount of details on and on and wearing her down with the intensity and negativity of the topic.

Much later in the conversation, she told me how she'd been feeling guilty about not being a good friend and supporting me when she knew I was struggling socially in downtown. In hindsight, I see that that was probably her big driver for inviting me up. I'd taken it as an invitation to pour my heart out and offload when maybe that was actually too much.

After that, we had a few awkward encounters—and one day at the mall where I was particularly overstimulated and grumpy—but then didn't see each other any longer. I got the feeling she was struggling with the urge to run, and so, in a state of dismay, I let her run. Perhaps I was too afraid to reach out and ask, "Do you still want to be friends with me?" It was sad, but I don't think she was really up to supporting someone as transitional and emotional as I was at the time.

And Angel—well, you know about that! I never did make full sense of Angel's reaction. Perhaps she was exhausted from her attempts to "fix" me and left with a feeling that it was all just too hard. I know that she was always focused on trying to help those in need. It was her Christian role and purpose, and she told me it was the reason she'd approached me in the first place. Perhaps she just wanted more gratitude and positivity from me.

I also wonder if there may have been some discrimination involved—not a nasty, I-won't-be-around-a-person-with-a-syndrome type of discrimination, just a slight, even subconscious, distaste at hearing I had a syndrome of some sort making her less eager to be around me. Or a sense of, "I give up. I don't want to be the one to have to deal with this person's social neediness." It would certainly be a hard thing for her to admit if so. But I can't make any assumptions one way or another. All I can say is these experiences were definitely bad.

So whatever the cause, losing these two friends at a time when I had almost nobody made me very on guard about the idea of telling anyone else about my Asperger's Syndrome, and I decided to sit on it for a while. I looked up the topic of telling other people about your Asperger's on online forums and found that others had had similar experiences. People wrote that the second you mention the word "Asperger's," neurotypical people put you in the "mental" category and don't really want to hang out with you. Many are not interested in understanding. They don't want to put in the work.

I argued that surely, being able to explain the syndrome would help people understand me better and aid communication with others. I had a daydream that when I told my friends, they would finally see where I was coming from and everything would become easier. The forum users wrote back that neurotypicals don't care. I was informed of a cold, hard reality.

Some months later, I tried again. I wrote a forum post about wanting to "come out of the Aspie closet" and explained that although it's illogical, the emotional side of me is still itching to tell people. I don't feel okay sitting on this secret. I need to be open and share this with those who are close to me.

Again, I got the same sorts of online responses. "It's a bad idea." Looking at all the replies, I started to see just how many Aspies out there have had awfully harsh experiences with typical people judging and dismissing them. One man wrote his story about how when he finally told his wife, she divorced him. It was one more thing on a long list of issues that had already been plaguing them. The label was the final straw.

So this is the place my mind was at when I began writing this book, talking about my secret that I carry with me. I reasoned that I had too much to lose by trying to talk to people about Asperger's and decided that not telling would be my default. Less risk of losing friends, full stop. Decision made. And in my rule-abiding way, I made the call and then put the concept out of my immediate thoughts.

But somewhere over time, it seems my opinion did gradually change, even though I wasn't consciously aware of it doing so. As my life went on, I started to meet and hear about people who were Aspies and wore the label proudly. My husband (at the time) mentioned to me a lawyer at his work who had introduced himself to the group as "the lawyer with Asperger's." He must have said it with confidence, because the general attitude toward him was respect and admiration of his talents.

There were a few guys in the League who also openly shared their Asperger's Syndrome with others in their lives without shame or any attempt to hide it. One guy in the group, Stephen, impressed me with his tendency to wear shirts with Asperger's-related humor or slogans. One of the first times I saw him in public, he was wearing a T-shirt that said, "I am not rude, hyper or weird. I have Asperger's Syndrome. What's your excuse?" And when I saw that, I thought how fantastic it was that he can walk around the shops and in public and not even care that others will see. He did it with confidence, and I'm now thinking that perhaps that's the key to success.

It doesn't matter what label you carry or what cause you stand for. If you approach the world with an assured attitude and pride in who you are, other people will love and respect you for it. It's only when you hide things about yourself that you convey that something is wrong or shameful about you that *needs* to be hidden. I guess this lesson just took me a year or two to learn.

Now that I think back, I wonder how many of those Aspies I saw on online forums were also lonely and hiding their Asperger's from the world. I'm guessing perhaps a lot, as the forums do attract a lot of new people who are just coming to terms with their condition, which would explain why the information I first received seemed to be so biased toward negative responses.

It's a shame that the sites don't attract more of those who are confident within themselves and wear their label with pride to be an example to others. But I suppose it's loneliness, frustration, and discontentedness that drive most people to these forums in the first place. It's hard to find the positive role models. They're too busy living their lives!

Anyway, one day more recently, I decided to redo an online Aspie quiz, just for fun, after seeing some of the other League members posting their results online. The test brought up my results:

Your Aspie score is 129/200

Your Neurotypical (Non Autistic) score is 68/200

You are very likely an Aspie.

And when I was looking at my results, it suddenly hit me . . .

I realized I don't care anymore if people know. I have enough friends now who know and accept me for who I am. I don't need to fear people walking away because of people's stereotypes and misunderstanding of what "Aspie" means. If they do, then they're not the people I really need in my life anyway.

I posted my quiz results on my main Facebook page and wrote exactly that. Just like that, I decided to come out of the Aspie closet. It was this momentous and amazingly bold thing to do! I couldn't believe I just did that!

Awaiting the results, at first, was quite stressful, and I hung back on Facebook, waiting to see what people would write in response. Would people write positive responses or just say nothing? Would anyone unfriend me? I hoped not. But overall, it was a move I'm so glad I made, because it allowed me to reach a point where I suddenly felt free and unburdened. Why had I been hiding myself from my friends for so long? I'm proud of who I am.

Fortunately, the replies that came weren't negative in any way. In fact, I got a few rather good responses to the post that I decided to copy here. Note that if the names look inconsistent, it's because I asked each individual how they wanted to be referred to. These are real people!

From an Aspie friend I met online, Cat Keller:

> Congrats on telling everyone!!!!!!
>
> Welcome to the world, from one Aspie to another!
>
> There is a secret to happiness . . . I was just sharing it with another Aspie. I'm going to share it with you, now that you're on the path to being truly happy and free . . .
>
> Just do you . . . just be Michelle . . . and fuck everything else, that's how I live. I just do Cat and I don't let what anyone else thinks have the least bit of influence.
>
> Come on out of the closet . . . everywhere.
>
> I wear the same outfit every day and the same night gown every night until they wear out and have to be replaced.
>
> I wash them, it's my business if I want to dress in the same thing.
>
> I don't have to choose my clothes, I know what I'm wearing.
>
> I say whatever comes to mind and I don't edit myself.
>
> I stopped trying to hide my tics.
>
> I do my rituals (OCD) and I'm not ashamed of them.
>
> Just let go and put it all out there—stop looking at how others react . . . just let them do them, and you do you . . . and happiness follows. We can't change that we're different, and the angst comes from wanting to, wanting to be like them . . . the day you let go of that, you'll find the world is a BEAUTIFUL place for you . . . and you can celebrate being different, as you should.
>
> Who the hell wants to be like everyone else?
>
> Frankly, I pity NT people.

The more eccentric, the more different, the more novel a person is . . . the more interesting they are to me.

NT people barely register on my radar.

Just do you.

Stop trying to hide behind learned behavior.

Do what feels natural.

Tic, blurt out what's in your head, stop trying to control where your hands want to be, quit living (or trying to live) by their rules—and watch the stress drain away.

You will find that people will love you for it will love you for being YOU.

It takes courage to let go and just be you at first, and after that, you won't believe you ever tried to do anything else.

It's the most freeing thing in the world.

No more hiding . . .

You've taken the first step on the path to happiness . . .

From one of my friends in Australia, Danielle:

> Yep, I agree, nothing wrong with being an Aspie! Everyone is so different in so many ways, it's just one way of looking at yourself and other people. Everyone has strengths and weaknesses, it's just one way of categorizing some of those typical characteristics! An Aspie that I know who realized as an adult said it just helped them to understand why they thought and acted differently to some people in certain situations, and it was empowering. :) I don't believe it changes who you are as a person—if we liked you before you had a 'label', it will be no different post-label. ;-)

From a friend who asked to remain anonymous:

> Wow what inspiring conversations you've got here Michelle! After reading all this I've come to the conclusion that no matter how hard I try, no matter how "much" I try, there will always be people who won't accept me for who I am. I'm never going to fit into their world per se. But reading all these comments brought a smile on my face. You've made me realize perhaps we're not all so different. I've

grown up thinking that it would all be so much easier if only I were "white," then I wouldn't get so many odd looks walking down the street as a kid. lol. (I grew up in Melbourne in the 80's where racism wasn't at its "subtle" stage, more like let's go pick on the poor Asian kid stage.) That unfortunately has tormented me and has made me realize that not only am I not "white," but I'm not "Asian" enough either to fit in with the new wave of Asian migrants. The fact that I couldn't fully understand why popular people were so popular didn't help. Luckily I've made friends with people who (thankfully!) genuinely like me. And without them I would be completely lost. I've only met you twice Michelle, and let me tell you, you ARE a beautiful woman and even if you don't think that at this point in time, well at least you've inspired me to rethink whether I feel the need to "fit in" all the time. On a different note, why do people like popular people??!

And last but not least, from a dear friend of mine I've known since high school, Daniel Scoullar:

Congratulations, Michelle, on the decision. I agree it is better to live your life authentically instead of hiding parts of yourself. Hiding yourself just leads to shame, whereas living courageously/honestly leads to pride. When you live openly and authentically, you will draw the people into your life who you need and who need you—and others will drift away. This is a hard process, but it leads to a good place. I hope this journey you are embarking on leads you to being connected to people who you can accept and love and who accept and love you in return. Life's too short for anything else. x

This final friend of mine is a strong advocate for lesbian, gay, bisexual, and transgendered rights, hence his references to pride and shame. It was this post that got me thinking again about the similarities between hiding one's Asperger's and hiding one's sexual preferences, and this train of thought that led me to write the next chapter.

Looking back, I like that this book is becoming a journey—a journey to me finding happiness, purpose, and confidence in being an adult with Asperger's Syndrome. I write about both the "now," learning to be proud of being an Aspie, and the "then," the story of where I've come from. And I'd like to dream that by the end of the book, I could become an inspiration for others like me to wear their Aspie with pride too. I want to celebrate this gift I've been given. I don't want to hide any more.

CHAPTER FIFTY-ONE

THE SIMILARITIES BETWEEN HAVING ASPERGER'S AND BEING LGBT

So, speaking about the LGBT community, it has occurred to me before that there are some interesting similarities between being an Aspie and being someone of non-typical gender or sexual identity. In both cases, we find ourselves stuck in an awkward position where who we are naturally is not yet fully accepted by society at large.

It puts so much pressure on us to hide a critical part of our makeup. For Aspies or transgendered people, this part is personality—who we are. For gay people, it's sexuality—who we're attracted to. In both cases, this part is *vital* and something we need to be able to show the world and celebrate to ever be truly proud of ourselves.

One of my Aspie friends, John Ronald, once wrote a post on Facebook where he eloquently described Aspies as "the natural allies to the LGBT" community, and I thought that was a nice way of seeing it. Both Aspies and LGBT people experience similar societal pressures, and we should be able to empathize with each other. For me, just considering showing the world my real self has been such a big transition from my old patterns of changing to fit in—or more specifically, acting "normal."

When I first began to understand that I had Asperger's Syndrome, I really did feel like it was a secret I needed to keep locked away for fear that others wouldn't understand. I was so afraid to lose friends over it if I dared expose the real and complete me. I'm so happy now to begin the process of coming out of the "Aspie closet." It's a new type of freedom!

I know that along the way, there may be some people who dismiss me for it. They may assume it means I'm mentally lacking and treat me accordingly, or they may talk about it as being just "excuses" for any non-typical behavior. But whatever they think, I guess I'm just going to have to ride through it, because I understand now that being proud of myself—all of me—is something I need if I ever really want to be happy and authentically me. And there is so much to be proud of!

For me, I love how being different has taught me to be a more compassionate and tolerant person. Wisdom and inner beauty don't come without life experience and some struggles, and I hope that in time, as the world grows and the culture changes, we will move toward a place where all people can be proud of who they are, whatever their unique qualities might be.

After all, it's differences that make us interesting and can create the most fascinating people—creative people and outside-of-the-box thinkers. What a boring world it would be if everyone was of the same normal, standard mold, the type that everyone is pressured to be growing up. What on Earth are we thinking in desiring that anyway?

CHAPTER FIFTY-TWO

MEETING OTHER ASPIES

Q: So, how did you go about meeting other Aspies? Was it a scary thing to do?

Yeah, you know, it was! So now we move on to the last chapter of my past story, which takes place only about six months before I started writing this book!

After my initial diagnosis, it took me many months to seek out and join any real-life Asperger's groups. Part of me really liked the idea of having a support group and being able to find like minds to socialize with. I wanted someone to discuss this diagnosis with. But I think part of me was still rejecting the idea that I could be like anyone with a label.

I made excuses to myself—the driving distance to the nearest group was just too far down an unfamiliar freeway. Driving the freeways of Texas wasn't something I was yet comfortable with. "It's too hard." I think the real reason I wasn't making the effort was that I was afraid of what I was going to find.

I recall having a discussion with Angel (actually, it was part of the last one-on-one discussion I ever had with her) in which I expressed my concerns that I didn't think I would fit in with other Aspies. I wasn't sure I wanted to go into the group among others who might be a lot more low-functioning than I was. Maybe deep down, it just sounded too confronting. I'm able to pass as normal, I told myself. I'm a competent person.

I didn't want to think of myself as being like these other Aspies I imagined up. It's disturbing how badly the media stereotype of Asperger's was ingrained in my head, and I really was vain enough to presume that I might be the only normal-seeming one.

However, despite my initial reservations, I jotted down some dates and locations of the closest Aspie meetup group in my diary and considered it for a while. Then, one particular month, I just decided, that's it, I'm going to make the effort to go to one of these things. And a heavily pregnant me jumped in the car and drove down to Sugarland, Texas for the first time. It turned out that with little traffic, the drive only took around twenty minutes. All those months of freeway fears had been completely unfounded.

My first meeting started out a little strange. I arrived a few minutes early and was ushered by a rather outgoing (no doubt neurotypical) young man to write my name down on a sign-in sheet and go sit at a row of chairs. I didn't realize it at first, but I'd been directed to the parents' section. I suppose being heavily pregnant and nicely dressed must have given too much of a "normal," parent-like impression for anyone to ask me my reasons for being there.

As usual, I felt uncomfortable sitting with the group of strangers and having to make small talk. There were periods of uncomfortable silence. I wanted the meeting to hurry up and start.

At one point, a guy approached the group (another adult Aspie, I was soon to find out). He was social and made funny jokes/banter that immediately put me at ease. His humor was spot on for me and struck a chord. I found myself grinning with genuine liking. Then he wandered off to talk to another group. And as that group walked together past the back of the parents' area and out of the room, I suddenly knew they were the adult Aspies.

I didn't know it because they were weird or embarrassing looking. It was more the feel the group gave me. They were characters, a collection of unique-looking people interacting in a close, friendly, open way. You could tell a few of them knew each other well. What wasn't there was that feeling of pretense and false enthusiasm—fakeness—that I usually get when I see a group of people talking.

These people weren't showing off or trying to be subtly better than each other. They weren't dressing to impress or giving off airs of importance. They were simply enjoying each other's company. All that, I got at a glance.

Suddenly, all that shallow, superficial crap just melted away. I wanted to go where that group of people was going. I wanted to know them. I asked one of the hosts who the group of people walking past were and where they were going. The host confirmed what I already knew. "That's the adult Asperger's group. They meet in a separate room over there." I explained that I was in the wrong place and excused myself.

Then off I went to join the adult group in the back room. I filled my name in on a sign-in sheet and took my place in a circle of chairs. There were only around ten to fifteen people in the room. It was so much more comfortable than the other group. I knew now that I was going to enjoy this meeting.

I don't remember what topics were covered in that first Aspie meeting, but I do remember walking away from it on a high, relieved and amazed to find so many people like myself. It was a mentally stimulating, meaningful, enjoyable conversation. I'd been craving that mental stimulation for so long. It had been badly lacking since I'd left work and had only social engagements to attend.

There were a few in the group whose behaviors were more outwardly challenged. They stood out. But for the most part, these people seemed outwardly "normal" too and comfortable to be around. I'd been completely misguided in my preconceived ideas about Aspies. More than that, these people felt safe to be around, completely safe and open. No airs required. I felt so comfortable being myself there, and I can't say I've ever experienced that to that level anywhere else. It was like coming home for the first time.

The group gathered socially at a restaurant after the meetup. I skipped the meal the first time but went to every one I could thereafter. I also joined various individual gatherings outside the main group.

A few months in, the League was created.

At one of our early League gatherings, I remember the group discussing the topic of acceptance versus belonging and how, for the first time for pretty much all of us, we suddenly felt like we were somewhere we really belonged.

To be "accepted" is to have other people tolerate you and allow you to join them in their various activities. Most of us had experienced some degree of this with our regular friends. However, to "belong" is to really feel like you're at the heart of the group, to have people value you and want you there. To know you're around "same."

I can't begin to express how experiencing a group like this changed my world and how it took away my need to try and be anything other than myself. Suddenly, I had friends and a social niche, and it didn't matter anymore what the rest of the world thought of me. I stopped trying so hard to fit where I just don't fit.

I began to attend the expatriate mums' groups less and less. I'd become busier now and no longer found it yielding when I had so many other things to do. From day one at that Aspie meeting, I felt more comfortable and connected with the people around me than some mums I had been trying to befriend for a year or more. The driver to keep fighting a losing battle was no longer there.

Other members of the League were expressing the same sorts of things:

David N. wrote:

> I got out of bed today and wished that I could sit and have some coffee and visit with my friends, the League of Extraordinary Aspies. I feel such a connection and sense of community with you, something I've never experienced before. A sense of belonging. I feel that I can truly be myself around you. I feel welcomed. I feel hopeful. I feel inspired! The NT world, by and large, has always been a frightening, troubling, uncertain, anxious, storm-tossed place for me. Thank you all so much, dear friends, for the haven of your fellowship.

ha·ven

noun

> **1.** a harbor or port.
>
> **2.** any place of shelter and safety, refuge, asylum.

John J. Ronald wrote (in response to David finding friends in the League):

> Glad it has helped, and I also feel that finally once again I've found a small circle of friends I can truly be myself around as well. It's been a LONG time since I felt that way . . .

My discussions with the League members also seemed to inspire me in amazing ways. Early on, one of the men in the group, David N., told me he found me so expressive and insightful and encouraged me to write it all down. Suddenly, I felt like people might actually want to hear what I had to say. I began writing this book and have been working on it ever since.

Another member of the League, Josh, was an inspired photographer. Looking at his nature pieces made me want to go out and photograph things too. That love of nature and eye for the beauty in my surroundings has always been in me. I'd considered studying or taking up photography before. Seeing it done so well flipped an "on" button for me, and I was suddenly in love with the world around me and had to go capture it on camera.

In a short time, I had more things I wanted to do than I possibly had time for. Not just wanted to do, but felt driven, *had* to do. Where had this buzz been all my life?

One day, it occurred to me why having a place in society made such an impact. It was because until now, I'd been depressed for most of my life. Being alone and alien to everyone around you leaves you wanting, and depression is a natural and common consequence of isolation.

Because I'd learned that other people don't like you when you act down, I had spent lengthy periods of my life suppressing it and acting "okay," at least until it got really bad. However, it was always there, with the exception of a few brief happy periods in life (early childhood, the end of high school, and some of my university and childcare studies).

Now, it was like a fog had been lifted. I wasn't just happy because there were things going on around me. I was happy because I was connecting to and belonging with people who valued the real me. I felt alive and wanted to explore who I was more and more and love myself more and more. Since I've found this side of me and seen so much beauty and value in what I can do, I can't imagine going back to feeling like I have no purpose anymore. Creating and sharing my life and learnings with others has become my purpose.

I am an Aspie, and I'm on a mission to show the rest of the world what a wonderful thing that is. I'm so proud to be an Aspie now that I see all the beautiful and brilliant things that come with it. It's the best gift life could have given me. I love spending time around other Aspies who share a common way of seeing things. I'm so happy to be me.

CHAPTER FIFTY-THREE

ASPIE HUMOR

Q: Do Aspies have a sense of humor?

No, we have absolutely no sense of humor at all. Full stop. (In case you can't tell there, I was being funny. Yet another winning, cringeworthy joke from me!) But before you throw down the book, I'll answer seriously.

I find it a strange thing how the media have created this running stereotype about Aspies being solemn, serious people who don't laugh at funny things or have any real sense of humor. I know where this idea comes from, but it couldn't be more wrong. Many of the adult Aspies I know have a fantastic sense of humor. We're quirky, witty, and creative in our banter, and I love the unique Aspie style.

I suppose the misunderstanding arises from the fact that Aspies and neurotypicals see humor in a very different way. We Aspies tell jokes that are a little out of the box, and typical people don't always immediately get it. They assume we're being weird instead of working out the meaning and realizing the humor. I guess some Aspie banter can require a little logical thinking to decipher.

Similarly, neurotypical people tell jokes that are figurative, and sometimes the younger, less experienced Aspies may not understand, giving them a rather aloof appearance. Inexperienced Aspies, particularly children or teens, also may fail to realize that when everyone else is laughing, the expected response is to smile and join in, even if you don't get it.

Such an Aspie could seem quite out of place looking serious, perhaps even frowning when concentrating to understand, in a laughing crowd. Some Aspies take things factually and may find figurative jokes hard to understand. I think most of us can understand them, but we come in all types.

However, it doesn't mean that Aspies are humorless and don't enjoy a good laugh. It simply means that what we find funny may be different than what you do.

Aspie humor itself can often be very literal. When I see signs saying, "End road work," I think, "Yes, road work is evil and must be stopped! Down with road work!" When I see a pedestrian crossing with lights and a sign saying, "Give way to cars when flashing," I get images of flashers trying to keep out of the way of motor vehicles (and a whole lot of amusing driver reactions that could go along with that!).

Some friends of mine started a running joke recently about the evil race of Ped Xing. Ped Xing are nasty creatures that commuters are frequently warned about on black-and-yellow street signs. The warning pictures depict a man with a detached head briskly walking as if to cross a road. Under the picture, the creature is labeled in clear black letters: "Ped Xing."

We understand that the Ped Xing are headless, zombie-like creatures that live by preying on the necks of regular humans to convert them to Ped Xing and further their race. They're neither alive nor dead. It's an epidemic, and they're spreading fast! In some areas, when you drive down the road, you'll see Ped Xing warning signs with flashing lights to warn you of major outbreaks in that area. In such places, it's crucial that you cover your neck and remain in your vehicle at all times.

Sometimes, a Ped Xing may be depicted with his wife or even headless children. These images may look cute—but be warned that it's only an illusion to draw you in. Even the Children Xing would have YOUR NECK in a second given the chance. Ped Xing are out there. People should beware!

Throughout this book, I have to say I haven't included *too* much outside-the-box humor, partly because the subject matter is serious anyway, but mainly because I can never be sure if the reader would completely get it or whether it would just create confusion. If you have no idea what I was going on about in those two paragraphs above, then this is a perfect example of what I mean. It's something I have to be careful about in real life too. I can't just assume people will be witty and random enough to catch on.

Face to face, I myself am quite a smiley, jovial sort of girl and take humor in many things, Aspie and neurotypical alike. I have enough awareness and life experience to follow most anything. But of all the humor in the world, nothing really entertains me like a good Aspie run of nonsensical information. Taking common rules or comments and applying them to things that just don't work. Making a statement that defines itself to be incorrect. Making a mockery of the way people use terms or phrases by applying them incorrectly. Throwing in ideas that are completely random for no reason, and linking all things back to previous inside jokes.

I love quirky humor. It's the best! And if you don't believe me, you can check with Ped Xing. He even has his own Facebook page![48] Go ahead. Log in. Friend him! He may not tell you the answer, but if he takes your neck, then at least that's one less person in the world who disagrees with me! Mwahahaha!

Of course, I'm kidding there. In real life, I don't actually go around killing or conspiring to kill people all that much. In fact, I'll admit it, I'm boring. I haven't been involved in killing any at all! I'm just a nerd who stays at home not murdering people in my free time. Lame, I know.

So, to finish off, here is an Aspie joke that a friend of mine wrote recently on Facebook and I just had to quote. It speaks for itself. Brilliant. Or at least I think so.

> A horse walks into a bar, and the Aspie bartender says, "Why the long face? You're a horse, so your face is physically long compared to that of a human, which is what I am. I'm asking like I want to know why you're depressed, but the truth is that the situation is more literal than one would expect."
>
> The horse didn't say anything, because horses can't talk.
>
> —Josh Mitchell

---

[48] http://www.facebook.com/ped.xing.33

CHAPTER FIFTY-FOUR

ADVICE FOR PARENTS

Q: What advice would you give to parents of children with Asperger's Syndrome?

Surprising as it may seem, I find this a rather hard question to answer, because as an Aspie myself, it's hard to imagine what it might be like for typical parents to raise a child on the spectrum.

I'm not familiar with their struggles and how a usual parent would see their Aspie child. But I do have some definite thoughts on what is important for the child. Back in March of 2011, I responded online to a similar question posted by the mother of a three-year-old boy with suspected Asperger's, and I think I covered it well then, so I'll paraphrase my answer here.

> Dear [Aspie mum],
>
> Firstly, I would say, something so important that many parents seem to forget is to make sure you give your son the self-esteem to deal with life and be happy with himself *as he is*, because he's going to experience at least some social rejection.
>
> We Aspies can learn to conform to varying degrees, but pushing us to change too much tends to make us unhappy, not happy, when it

gets to the point where we no longer feel it is okay to be ourselves. And any bullying we receive in school or out in the world is going to make us even less self-confident. So yes, do teach him social skills, but don't push him too hard. Teach him that he's wonderful as he is, and focus on his gifts.

In answer to your question about my experiences, yes, I'm an Aspie myself, but I only found out in my late twenties, and I think my life would have been very different if I'd had someone teaching me self-acceptance and encouraging me to flourish as I was.

Unfortunately for us "missed generation," a lot of us weren't diagnosed young, so there was little help, understanding, or acceptance around when we grew up, just expectations. People didn't make allowances for our differences, and we didn't have the advantage that your children are going to have.

I wish the best for your son, and if any of my children ever turn out to be AS, I plan on giving them the best positive start I can.

Kind regards,

Michelle

CHAPTER FIFTY-FIVE

KNOWING IF YOU ARE AN ASPIE

Q: I actually have a few Aspie-like characteristics myself. How would I be able to tell if I was an Aspie?

Knowing you're an Aspie isn't something that just happens the second you stumble across it. I think many of us who discover it for ourselves have long periods of questioning and even denial at first.

It's an odd and unbelievable concept to take in that you yourself could be someone different from the norm. Unthinkable.

I remember my thoughts chopping and changing frequently for those first several months after I really looked into it. One week I would be thinking, "Maybe I am an Aspie. It just all seems to fit." The next, "No, I'm normal. What was I thinking?" Then another discovery or discussion I read would prompt me to think, "Oh, wow! Maybe I really am!" all over again. And so it went on.

I think the reason it takes us so long is because Aspie behavior isn't an easy thing for a person to see in themselves. Even when our differences are great, they may not stand out to us Aspies because we're so used to them being our "normal." We have no experience at being anyone else and don't perceive ourselves from other people's points of view. (Theory of mind is not exactly our strong point!)

However, reading about Asperger's from the point of view of real Aspies is a great way to slowly see it clearly. I started my journey thinking, "Maybe I have a little bit of this," and read on with curiosity. The more I read, the more it just became apparent that I really *am* this. It was a case of "everything fits." After a while, I reached a point where it was undeniable, and "Aspie" began to feel like part of my identity. Now I can't imagine myself as anything else.

If you suspect that you yourself are an Aspie, it's quite possible you may be or at least have something with overlapping symptoms. Just the questioning makes me think something is going on, because typical people don't really tend to ponder these things. They don't relate to our idiosyncrasies. In this case, the best thing you can do is learn more! From books and articles to online forums and adult Aspie community groups, there's a lot of information out there.

One easy way to get a better indicator of how likely you are to be an Aspie is to take an online Aspie quiz. They're easy to find if you Google words like "Aspie," "Quiz," "Autism," etc. However, keep in mind that these tests are only indicative.

Another method I found personally helpful was reading through lists of questions that an Aspie might answer yes to or agree with, such as:

- I frequently get so strongly absorbed in one thing that I lose sight of other things.

- I tend to have very strong interests, which I get upset about not being able to pursue.

- Have you felt different from others for most of your life?

- Do you or others think that you have unconventional ways of solving problems?

- Do people see you as eccentric?

- Do you have a strong eye for detail?

- As a child, was your play more directed toward, for example, sorting, building, investigating, or taking things apart than toward social games with other kids?

- In a social group, it can be difficult to keep track of several different people's conversations.

And many, many more! I've included a rather extensive list of questions in Appendix Two if you'd like to keep reading further examples.

Then, of course, if you really just have to know or you feel that you're in need of help, there's always the option of a formal diagnosis.

For some of us, having that label after so many years of not knowing can be a great relief. For others, it's unnecessary and unappealing to be categorized. Either way, as a grown adult, don't feel that diagnosis is compulsory if you're functioning perfectly fine as you are. It's your choice. Diagnosed, undiagnosed, questioning, or just interested on behalf of a loved one or friend, the Aspie community is pretty welcoming to everyone.

Chapter Fifty-Six

What's Next for Me?

Well, isn't that the big question! Right now, I think I'm in a pretty good place in life and have lots of funny little ideas and daydreams that I'd like to pursue in the future. Many of these are ideas that excite me and make me want to get up and go each day. It's certainly a different place than where I've been in the past.

I've been finding a lot of joy in dabbling in photography (and even more so the editing), and I like to imagine having more time to play with that. I'd love it if one day I could get a macro lens and take pictures of bugs up close—creepy to most, I know, but that would be so very me! I've even considered getting involved in stock photography if I ever find the time. Being able to make a little money out of something I love would be a positive way of achieving independence. But we'll see how that goes.

On the work front, I think I still feel a little too troubled from my past experiences to really consider a formal job again, at least in the traditional way. However, if something right for me ever fell into my lap that allowed me the freedom I need to do things my way, then I could be open to it. I do love planning and scheduling things. Maybe someone could pay me to organize elements of other people's lives or businesses! Just the bits that you do on paper. That might be fun, though I've never heard of a job exactly in that field!

I also discovered recently how much fun I have editing sound files, so maybe that's something else I could look into one day. Again, if I find the time.

On the Asperger's front, I have many thoughts that inspire me. I feel passionate about communicating to people what Asperger's really is and what we really need. I'd like to encourage society at large to be more accommodating of us, especially in the workforce, and not just focus on training us to slot in with them. Maybe one day, I could advocate for Asperger's and/or go around answering questions on the topic. (Presuming it's not too scary to do so!) I imagine publishing this book could be a great way to initiate that.

I'm happy the League has been started, and I would encourage more such social groups around the world. As an Aspie, the difference it makes to have other like people as friends can't be emphasized enough. Currently, our group has been dwindling in numbers as people come and go, but I'd like to see it going strong again.

Earlier in the year, we were toying with making podcasts of our Aspie-centered discussions. It would be great if we could pick that up again and turn it into something regular and presentable for all the isolated Aspies out there to listen to and know they're not alone.

Most exciting, I think, are the daydreams that I have in regard to writing this book. It's impossible, really, for me to guess how a reader might find my writing. Is it unique and insightful enough to be interesting to a typical person, or will they just see it as boring, boring, boring? I can't imagine reading it from someone else's point of view. But I'm determined to try, because there's so much I wish for people to understand.

I want people to see how, if we Aspies were utilized better, what amazing things we could contribute and how much untapped talent is currently wasting away behind social barriers and difficulties. I want businesses to realize that it requires a certain accommodation of our needs and level of freedom before an Aspie can spread their wings and fly, and we need more opportunities to fly!

It's possible that this book will never take off as I wish, but I'd like to at least hope that my unique views and experiences will be of interest to the psychological community and/or to other adults with Aspies in their own lives. Even better, I like to daydream that the book might be an interesting story in itself that people would want to share with their typical friends. I could become an "author."

If I let myself get really carried away, I might sit and stare into space, fantasizing about being added to popular book club reading lists. (Come on, Oprah, help me out here!) I take delight in imagining it making high school reading curriculum or being recommended on television shows. It would be a book to educate teenagers about tolerance and accepting others who are different from themselves.

I daydream about how it could be marketed and the various words that could be written on the back cover. I imagine people sharing it around on Facebook and other social media and it becoming a well-known title. I would love to be remembered as someone who made great strides toward helping the high-functioning Autism community become understood by the world and getting people to take an interest in knowing more.

Maybe there could be something special about me once again.

Okay, I know that I really am fantasizing now. I have a way of coming up with daydreams and just can't help being carried away by the amazing high of all the outcomes I can imagine. It makes me feel like I'm flying—soaring in the air, delirious with happiness. I know it's unrealistic. I know much of this may never eventuate.

Oh, but I do love to dream . . .

APPENDIX ONE

	FEMALE BRAIN	MALE BRAIN
White matter (connecting tissue)	More[1]	Less
Corpus Callosum (interconnecting structure between brain hemispheres)	20% larger than male[3]	Less
Grey matter (processing tissue)	Less dense	More densely developed than that of women[5]
Brain size	Slightly smaller	Slightly larger
Amygdala Center for emotional reactions. (Fight and flight). Signals from the amygdala bypass the frontal lobe (rational thinking) and trigger rapid reactions.	Normal	Normal
Cerebellum (motor activity)	Normal	Normal
Frontal lobe (rational thinking)	Normal	Normal

THE AUTISTIC BRAIN

AUTISTIC BRAIN	MEANING
Less	Women can transfer data between the two sides of the brain faster than men[2] and use both sides of the brain more evenly.
Significantly smaller than that of a typical person[4]	Autistic people may have difficulties shifting information from one area of the brain to another. Women are naturally better at things like multitasking, subtleties in communication, verbal abilities, empathizing, etc.
Increased grey matter volume[6]	Men are naturally better at things like logic, systemizing, problem solving, spacial awareness and mental rotation of objects
Increased brain volume	Autistic people have less information transfer, and more reliance on singular hemisphere processing. Tendency towards hyperfocus.
Studies are inconclusive. More densely packed but small and immature cells	?? Aspies do appear more able to continue logical thinking in times of emotional crisis. During social evaluation tests Autistic subjects used the Amygdala less and relied on the Frontal lobe more (rational thinking brain)[9]
Larger in people with Autism[7] But possible decreased connectivity within[8]	?? Unsure. Could be linked to Autistic tendency towards poor gross motor skills
Increased local cortical connectivity,[10] increased cortex volume,[11] and increased concentration of metabolites found[12]	More ability for intense logical thinking. Local, rather than global (brain) information processing.

References:

1, 5. Haier, Richard et. al., "The neuroanatomy of general intelligence: sex matters", NeuroImage, Volume 25, Issue 1, Pages 320–327, March 2005, quoted in: Carey, Bjorn. 'Men and Women Really Do Think Differently.' LiveScience. Jan. 20, 2005. http://www.livescience.com/health/050120_brain_sex.html

2. Grey, Dr. John, 'The Male vs. the Female Brain', ThirdAge.com, April 27, 2011, http://www.thirdage.com/love-romance/the-male-vs-the-female-brain

3. Gurian, M. (2001). 'Boys and girls learn differently!: A guide for teachers and parents'. San Fransico, CA: Jossey-Bass., page 27

4. Egass, B., et. al., "Reduced size of corpus callosum in autism", Arch Neurol., 52(8):794-801, August 1995, http://www.ncbi.nlm.nih.gov/pubmed/7639631

6. Harden, Antonio, et. al., "An MRI Study of Increased Cortical Thickness in Autism", Am J Psychiatry., 163(7): 1290–1292, July 2006, http://www.ncbi.nlm.nih.gov/pmc/articles/PMC1509104/

7. Piven, Joseph, et.al., "An MRI study of autism: The cerebellum revisited", Neurology, Vol 49 no.2, Pp 546-551, August 1 1997, http://www.neurology.org/content/49/2/546

8. Mostofsky, Stewart, et. Al., "Decreased connectivity and cerebellar activity in autism during motor task performance", Brain (A Journal of Neurology), Volume 132, Issue 9, Pp. 2413-2425, September 2009, http://brain.oxfordjournals.org/content/132/9/2413.abstract

9. Ashwin C, Baron-Cohen S, Fletcher P, Bullmore E, Wheelwright S 2001 fMRI study of social cognition in people with and without autism. (International Meeting for Autism Research abstr B-32), quoted in: Amaral, David G., et al., 'The Amygdala, Autism and Anxiety', Foundation Symposium 251, Autism: Neural Basis and treatment possibilities, June 2002, http://psych.colorado.edu/~munakata/csh/Novartis_paper_6-12-02.doc

10. Murias, Michael et. al., "Resting state cortical connectivity reflected in EEG coherence in individuals with autism", Biol Psychiatry; 62(3): 270–273, August 1 2007, http://www.ncbi.nlm.nih.gov/pmc/articles/PMC2001237/

11. Carpenter, Ruth et. al., "Inverse correlation between frontal lobe and cerebellum sizes in children with autism", Brain (A Journal of Neurology), 123 (4): 836-844, 2000, http://brain.oxfordjournals.org/content/123/4/836.short

12. Murphy, et al., "Asperger Syndrome: A Proton Magnetic Resonance Spectroscopy Study of Brain," Arch. Gen. Psychiatry, 59:885-891, 2002, http://faculty.washington.edu/chudler/asp.html

Appendix Two

Questions an Aspie Might Answer Yes to or Agree With

These questions were collected from multiple Internet sources, most notably RDOS.[49]

- I frequently get so strongly absorbed in one thing that I lose sight of other things.

- I tend to have very strong interests, and I feel upset if I can't pursue them.

- Have you felt different from others for most of your life?

- Do you or others think that you have unconventional ways of solving problems?

- Do you have values and views that are either very old fashioned or way ahead of their time?

- Do people see you as eccentric?

- Do you have a strong eye for detail?

---

[49] http://www.rdos.net/eng/aspeval/relf1.htm

- As a child, was your play more directed toward, for example, sorting, building, investigating, or taking things apart than toward social games with other kids?

- In a social group, it can be difficult to keep track of several different people's conversations.

- Do you need periods of contemplation?

- People sometimes tell me that I keep going on and on about the same thing.

- Do you have an avid perseverance in gathering and cataloguing information on a topic of interest?

- Do you have strong sense of ethics and a tendency to stand up for your ideals and beliefs?

- Do you tend to do everything worth doing more perfect than really needed?

- Do you have one or a few special talents which you have emphasized and worked on?

- Do you consider yourself a very logical person?

- If there's an interruption, it takes me time to switch back to what I was doing.

- Are your thoughts persistent?

- Do you like to get lost in thought?

- Do you often work through lunch or breaks to fix mistakes and get things done on time?

- I would rather go to a library than to a party.

- Are you very logical and get surprised or impatient when others aren't?

- Do you enjoy figuring out how things work?

- Do you have excellent long-term memory in subjects that interest you?

- Do you have extraordinary abilities and deficits?

- Do you prefer to try to find your own niche in work/life?

- Are you determined to seek the truth?

- I tend to notice details that others do not.

- Are you irritated by inefficiency and do you find it easy to see how things can be done in better ways?

- Are you a complex person?

- Do you often feel out of sync with others?

- Do you avoid crowds?

- Are you disinterested in what is currently in vogue?

- Do you more often get things because you need them than because others have them?

- Is your sense of humor different from mainstream or considered odd?

- Do you see your own activities as more important than other people's?

- Do your feelings cycle regularly between hopelessness and extremely high confidence?

- Do you find it easier to understand & communicate with computers, animals, and/or Aspies than with "ordinary" people?

- Do you have a tendency to become stuck when asked questions in social situations?

- Do you have more difficulties than others of the same age when it comes to making friendships and getting into relationships?

- Do you find yourself more attracted to things, ideas, music, computers, animals, buildings, or vehicles than to people and social exchange?

- Do you tend to feel nervous, shy, confused, or left out in social situations?

- Do you avoid talking face-to-face with someone you don't know very well?

- Do you prefer to avoid eye-contact?

- Do you get very tired after socializing and need to regenerate alone?

- Do people think you are aloof and distant?

- Are you more of an observer than one who participates in life?
- Do you mostly prefer to play/work/do things on your own—in your own way and at your own pace?
- Do you prefer animals to people?
- Do you prefer to be alone?
- Do you mostly talk when you have something concrete to say?
- Do you often have lots of thoughts that you find hard to verbalize?
- In conversations, do you need extra time to carefully think out your reply, so there may be a pause before you answer?
- Do you often not know where to put your arms?
- Do you tend to talk either too softly or too loudly?
- Do you prefer to do things the same way over and over again?
- Have you been accused of staring?
- Do you rehearse inside your head?
- Do you have a habit of repeating your own or others' last words, internally or out loud (echolalia)?
- People occasionally comment that my conversation is confusing.
- I don't usually notice small changes in a situation or a person's appearance.
- Do others often misunderstand you when you act naturally?
- Do you find it difficult to figure out how to behave in various situations?
- Do you have problems with timing in conversations?
- When I talk on the phone, I'm not sure when it's my turn to speak.
- Other people frequently tell me that what I've said is impolite, even though I think it is polite.
- Do you sometimes not feel anything at all, even though other people expect you to?
- In conversations, do you tend to focus on your own thoughts rather than on what your listener might be thinking?
- I find myself drawn more strongly to things than people.

- Is being honest so natural to you that you often don't notice— or care—if others may find your remarks inappropriate, hurtful, or rude?

- People often tell me that I went too far in driving my point home in a discussion.

- Do you have a fascination with flowing water?

- Are you easily overexcited, stressed, and overwhelmed by things like noise, crowds, clutter, patterns, flicker, and movement?

- I sometimes find that I don't know how to keep a conversation going.

- Do you have difficulties filtering out background noise when talking to someone?

- Do you dislike when people walk behind you?

- When I was young, I wasn't very interested in games involving pretending with other children.

- Has it been harder for you than for others to keep friends?

- Do you find it stressful to go to a new place alone for the first time?

- Do you have difficulty accepting criticism, correction, and direction?

- I usually notice car number plates or similar strings of information.

- Are you sometimes afraid in safe situations, yet fearless in situations which may actually be dangerous?

- Do you easily get frustrated and upset when you're stressed, tired, hungry, interrupted, questioned, over-stimulated, or when things don't go as you had anticipated?

- Have you had a tendency to prefer the company of those who are older or younger than yourself?

- I often notice small sounds when others do not.

- Have you had the feeling of playing a game, pretending to be like people around you?

- Do you feel that people are watching you?

- Do you dislike discussing a topic that may not be of primary interest?

- I like to carefully plan any activities I participate in.

ABOUT THE AUTHOR

Michelle Vines was born in Liverpool, Australia and grew up in a hilly forest region of Melbourne known as the Dandenong Ranges. After showing talent in the areas of mathematics and science, Michelle was accepted into the University of Melbourne where she received bachelor's degrees with honors in chemical engineering and environmental science. Michelle began her career as a process engineer in the oil and gas industry and subsequently became a technical leader in manufacturing. However, after five years of feeling deeply unhappy in her work environment, Michelle paused her engineering career in 2008.

In 2010, Michelle moved to the United States with her one-year-old son, where she had another son the following year. She gradually grew to love the town of Houston, Texas, and has chosen to remain ever since.

At thirty years old, on the advice of friends, Michelle approached a psychologist at the University of Texas Health Science Center for assessment and was officially diagnosed with Asperger's syndrome. Michelle found the diagnosis to be a huge relief, and she has since dedicated a lot of her time to advocating for people on the Autism spectrum with the goal of helping the general public better understand the Autistic person's perspective. In 2013, she gave a public presentation on "Life as an Adult with Asperger's Syndrome," which has been viewed by tens of thousands of people on YouTube and has been instrumental in giving many others hope and the courage to seek out their own Asperger's diagnosis.

CONNECT WITH MICHELLE

EMAIL:	michellevines1980@gmail.com
FACEBOOK:	facebook.com/Michelle.Vines.31
TWITTER:	@AspieOTInside
YOUTUBE:	youtube.com/user/mvic80

GREY GECKO PRESS

Thank you for reading this book from Grey Gecko Press, an independent publishing company bringing you great books by your favorite new indie authors.

Be one of the first to hear about new releases from Grey Gecko: visit our website and sign up for our New Release or All-Access email lists. Don't worry: we hate spam, too. You'll only be notified when there's a new release, we'll never share your email with anyone for any reason, and you can unsubscribe at any time.

At our website you can purchase all our titles, including special and autographed editions, preorder upcoming books, and find out about two great ways to get free books, the Slushpile Reader Program and the Advance Reader Program.

And don't forget: all our print editions come with the ebook free!

www.GreyGeckoPress.com

SUPPORT INDIE AUTHORS & SMALL PRESS

If you liked this book, please take a few moments to leave a review on your favorite website, even if it's only a line or two. Reviews make all the difference to indie authors and are one of the best ways you can help support our work.

Reviews on Amazon, GreyGeckoPress.com, GoodReads, Barnes and Noble, or even on your own blog or website all help to spread the word to more readers about our books, and nothing's better than word-of-mouth!

http://smarturl.it/review-aspergers

RECOMMENDED READING

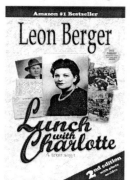
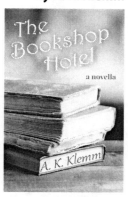

CPSIA information can be obtained
at www.ICGtesting.com
Printed in the USA
LVOW12*0507210318
570587LV00002B/8/P

9 781938 821950